BREAK FREE
FROM THE
SUGAR
BLUES

JANET SANDERS, J.D., C.H.C.

CAUTIONARY NOTE: Break Free from the Sugar Blues and the Sugar-Free Lifestyle Roadmap™ are designed to promote awareness about cutting sugar as well as blood sugar and diabetes control and to provide information, tools, and techniques that will enable individuals to make healthy lifestyle choices.

The coaching techniques are not intended to replace medical advice or to address any individual's specific medical problem(s). Always seek the advice of a physician before beginning any diet, exercise, or nutritional program. Diabetes and pre-diabetes are serious medical conditions. Program participants should not reduce, change, or discontinue any medication or treatment without consulting their physician.

You should also consult with your physician about food choices you would like to make in the context of your state of health or treatment plan. This is critical if you are taking any medications. Changing your eating patterns can lead to lower blood sugar levels, and you need to avoid having blood sugar levels drop too low. You should work with your medical provider to manage medications appropriately.

The materials in Break Free from the Sugar Blues do not replace professional help for mental health care. If you are experiencing anxiety, depression, or an eating disorder that requires professional care, reach out to a mental health care provider. If you are experiencing extreme depression or having suicidal thoughts, seek assistance from a professional ASAP.

©2025, Janet Sanders, All Rights Reserved. (Copyright ID: 1-15037154821)

No part of this book may be reproduced, stored in a retrieval system, or transmitted by any means without the written permission of the author.

Paperback ISBN: 978-0-9747573-1-5

Hardcover ISBN: 978-0-9747573-2-2 e-book ISBN: 978-0-9747573-3-9

Published by Great Life, Inc.

October, 2025

Ardmore, PA

DEDICATION

Break Free from the Sugar Blues is dedicated to the millions of people who struggle with conquering sugar and blood sugar health issues such as insulin resistance, pre-diabetes, diabetes, constant cravings, and yo-yo weight gain.

If you have tried a diet plan or education program in the past and continue to find yourself going off track, here is why:

- It doesn't matter if it is the greatest diet in the world.
- It doesn't matter if it has lots of delicious recipes or fabulous advice.
- No diet or food plan will work if you can't stick with it.

Break Free from the Sugar Blues is a comprehensive blueprint for change that I wish I had been given years ago when I first started addressing my compulsion to eat cookies, sweets, and other foods that led to my diagnosis of type 2 diabetes.

I am certain it would have spared me from years of uncontrolled sugar consumption, yo-yo dieting, and frustration, and I am confident that it will show you how to eliminate the roadblocks holding you back so that you can stop struggling and live a life you love.

Whether you are new to all of this or looking to get back on track, you are about to begin a journey of self-exploration that will provide you with the opportunity to change your life. I am here for you with practical solutions, coaching, and support every step of the way.

Thank you to everyone who helped me bring this book into the world. A message of gratitude goes to my friend, teacher, and mentor, Judith Cassis, who is no longer with us. I could not have done this without her coaching and support. Alishonn Bonnet (Shonn) and Kharisma Ozuna, I am grateful for your assistance with my book cover and editing. Nada Qamber, your amazing design work turned my words and pictures into a publication that brings my coaching to life.

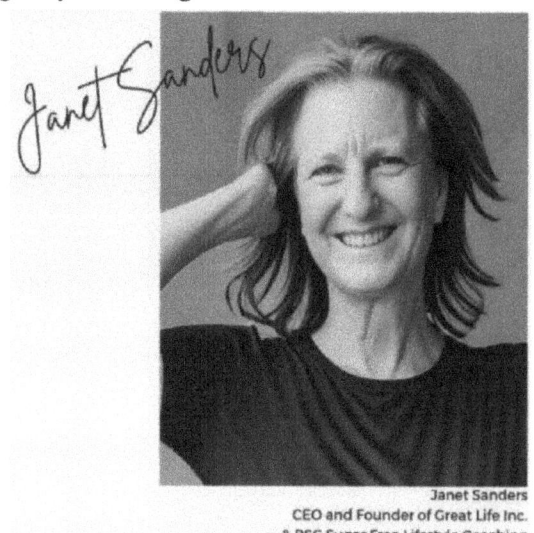

Janet Sanders
CEO and Founder of Great Life Inc.
& BSC Sugar Free Lifestyle Coaching

A special thanks to Tony Adler, Zack Smith, Jessica Mathews, and the entire team at Wiz Publishing for your assistance and encouragement during the final stages of the publishing process.

To my family, who have encouraged me throughout the years, nothing means more to me than your love and support. You helped me cross the finish line, and I am eternally grateful.

CONTENTS

DEDICATION   I

PREFACE   1

CHAPTER 1 The Struggle with Sugar Is Real   2

INTRODUCTION: Why Is Quitting Sugar So Hard?   11

CHAPTER 2 Sugar Consumption is on the Rise   12

THE SUGAR, MIND, AND BODY CONNECTION   18

CHAPTER 3 Eating Food Is Enmeshed in Every Aspect of Our Life   19

CHAPTER 4 Changing Your Relationship with Sugar   21

HOW TO USE THIS BOOK TO ACHIEVE RESULTS   30

CHAPTER 5 The Roadmap to Sugar-Free Vibrant Health   31

CHAPTER 6 Coaching Tips for Success   36

PHASE ONE: Embrace Change to Break Free from Sugar   40

CHAPTER 7 Commit to Making Lasting Changes and Adopting the 4 C's Of Change   41

CHAPTER 8 Connect to Yourself and a Supportive Community to Let Go of the Past   51

CHAPTER 9 Consistently Take Action to Quit Sugar and Adapt to a Sugar-Free Lifestyle   59

CHAPTER 10 Gain Clarity (Where You Are and Where You Want to Go) to Embark on a New Beginning   **84**

PHASE TWO: Nourish Your Body to Live Free from Sugar   **117**

CHAPTER 11 Learn How Your Body Works: The Sugar, Mind, and Body Connection   **118**

CHAPTER 12 Implement a Food Plan that Eliminates Personal Trigger Foods   **152**

CHAPTER 13 Validate, Monitor, and Adjust Your Plan   **210**

CHAPTER 14 Enhance Your Food Plan with Exercise, Restful Sleep, and Stress Management   **219**

PHASE THREE: Transform Your Mind to Stay Free from Sugar   **247**

CHAPTER 15 Find the Thoughts, Roadblocks, and Eating Patterns Getting in Your Way   **248**

CHAPTER 16 Reverse Sabotaging Thoughts, Habits, and Eating Patterns   **260**

CHAPTER 17 Eliminate Clutter in Your Space to Create an Environment that Supports Lasting Change   **288**

CHAPTER 18 Enjoy Life   **303**

COMING FULL CIRCLE: The 4 C's Of Change and Resilience   **307**

APPENDIX A: COACH & COOK GUIDE   **308**

APPENDIX B: SUGGESTED READING AND RESOURCES   **339**

APPENDIX C: WORKSHEETS   **342**

PREFACE

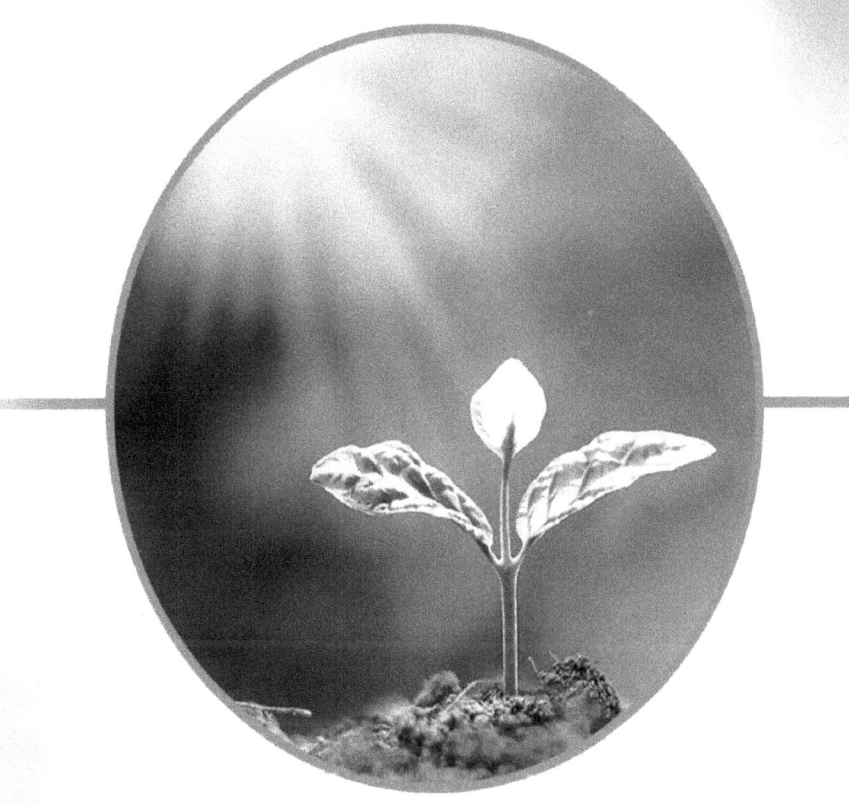

No matter how hard the past,
you can always begin again.
The Buddha

CHAPTER 1
The Struggle with Sugar Is Real

Millions of people worldwide wake up every day with a strong intention to kick sugar to the curb and still go to bed wondering what went wrong. Individual reasons for quitting sugar may be different, but the struggle is the same.

For some people, the driving force to quit sugar is exhaustion from yo-yo weight gain and years of unsuccessful dieting. Emotional eating can also fuel a love-hate relationship with sugar that is as gut-wrenching as any other out-of-control addiction.

If you have been beating yourself up because you find sugar getting the best of you, I am here to tell you that you can put your fists down. You are about to learn how to eat in harmony with how your body works and how to eliminate the roadblocks and trigger foods keeping you stuck. If you are new to all of this, *Break Free from the Sugar Blues* will guide you toward a new way of eating and living a sugar-free lifestyle.

The Day that Changed My Life

My journey to go sugar-free began with the diagnosis of type 2 diabetes in September 2001. It was a day that changed my life forever, and I remember the call from my doctor's office as if it were yesterday. As I listened to the nurse tell me that I had type 2 diabetes, I struggled to absorb her words. She tried to reassure me that everything would be fine, but she did not grasp that my world was turning upside down.

I hung up the phone and went upstairs to have a good cry. I wasn't sad; I was incredibly angry. The crazy thing was that although diabetes complications scared me, I was even more frightened by the thought of living my life without sugar. Food was my coping mechanism, and I had no idea how I could get through even a single day without eating the cookies, bread, cake, candy, pasta, and potatoes that literally were my lifeline to sanity. Up in my bedroom, I fell onto my bed and just started screaming, "I'M SO MAD, I'M SO PISSED OFF, I DON'T WANT TO HAVE DIABETES!" Finally, exhaustion took over, and my screams gave way to sobbing—sobbing to quiet weeping. My poor dog didn't know what to do. He jumped onto the bed and licked my face, trying to get me to cheer up. I curled up in a ball with my furry friend, and a sense of calm took over.

I don't think the anger ever really goes away, especially once you learn that type 2 diabetes is something that could have been avoided. But once my crying jag was over, I decided not to be a victim and to take control of my situation. I hugged my dog, got out of bed, and went downstairs to make dinner. For the last time, I ate whatever I wanted without worrying about my blood sugar.

My Love Affair with Sugar

My sugar-free journey started in 2001, but my love affair with sugar began when I was a young girl living with my very intelligent but crazy, alcoholic parents, who raised six children with the help of a house full of staff who kept us fed, clothed, and out of trouble. Food was a mainstay of our lifestyle, from lavish parties to family celebrations, midnight snacks, and afternoon treats.

One particular day, when I was 4 years old, provides some insight into the beginnings of my obsession with sweets and cookies. I do not know why the snippet of a day over 60 years ago is embossed in my mind with such clarity. But to this day, I can see myself through a time tunnel as if it were yesterday. I had just arrived home from nursery school, and as he did every day, the driver of the school's white van pulled into the large circular driveway, opened the exit door, and handed me two small cookies before I stepped out. The cookies were round and filled with icing, a 1950s version of my precious Oreos.

It was a perfect afternoon. The sun was shining, and as soon as my patent leather shoes touched the ground, I felt the warm asphalt under my feet and the wind blowing through my hair. A mysterious veil of happiness unfurled around me, imprinting a sense of bliss in my brain for reasons a 4-year-old could not possibly understand.

Walking towards the house, I slowly took little bites out of my cookies until both were gone. As I entered the house, the magic moment disappeared, waiting to be called upon many times throughout my life when a bit of magic was what my soul needed.

I Would Kill for a Cookie!

Fast-forward to 1988. I was a newly married attorney working in a Philadelphia law firm on one of the biggest fire disaster cases in the United States. I had my eye on the partnership prize, but there was just one little problem. The stress of my job and daily compulsive eating were literally destroying my insides.

One summer afternoon, as I was rushing out to grab a soda, I passed by the window of a local bookstore. A book with a really big cookie on the cover caught my eye. The title almost took the wind out of me: "I'd Kill for a Cookie: A Simple Six-Week Plan to Conquer Stress Eating." If books could talk, they would have called out my name. Stress eating, especially cookies, is my life story! I had been eating cookies to calm my nerves from the time I was a little girl through adulthood, when cookies and sugar saw me through college, law school, raising children, and working as a Philadelphia lawyer. I immediately ran inside, bought the book, and returned to my office, where I closed the door and read it from cover to cover. For the first time, a little ray of hope appeared that told me I was on to something, that maybe I could ditch the cookies and all the other sugary foods I consumed every day.

Finding this book was a beginning, but shaking sugar turned into a chaotic journey with lots of stops and starts. After reading the book, I tried for a few years to get my health in order with one diet after another, but no diet ever lasted very long. I was the queen of yo-yo weight gain, which finally came to an end in 2001 when I could no longer hide from the reality of my situation. It seemed like a disaster, but diabetes was the gift that finally saved my life. They say that insanity is doing the same thing over and over and expecting a different result. I knew I had to do things differently.

My Unlikely Transition to Health Coaching

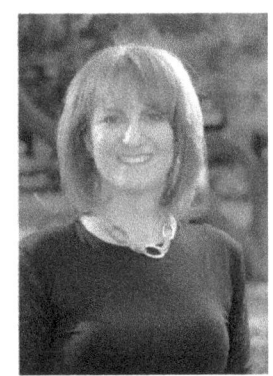

My transition to health coaching was not an initial part of my life plan. But once the reality of diabetes set in, I found myself at a crossroads. I stepped back from the stress of litigation and began to focus on helping legal organizations improve their processes for more effective litigation outcomes. It occurred to me that maybe I could apply the same principles I had used in the business world to make needed changes in my own life.

The lightbulb went on! I discovered that quitting sugar and healing my body was not just about what I was eating but more about what was "eating" me. I needed to learn how to navigate the changes that were happening to me and how to let go of the past. Most importantly, I had to figure out how to transform my mind so that I could cope with life's challenges without turning to food for comfort, while also nourishing my body in a way that put an end to the constant physical cravings for sugar.

My immediate mission was to:

- Think about my health in a new way,
- Gain the information I needed to make informed lifestyle decisions, and
- Successfully implement lifestyle changes that would last a lifetime.

As part of my journey, I found two books that ignited my transformation. The first was "Transitions, Making Sense of Life's Changes" by William Bridges, and the second was a gem of a book called "The Art of Getting Well" by David Spero. I devoured their contents and applied this new knowledge to the techniques that I had mastered as an attorney, project manager, and change management consultant.

I spent a year working with a doctor specializing in integrative medicine, taking cooking classes, studying nutrition, and developing coaching techniques while at the same time applying the principles I was learning to my own recovery. Once I put my plan into action, the insulin resistance fueling my chronic high blood sugars and yo-yo weight gain disappeared, and I was on the road to recovery. In six months, I lost over thirty pounds, reduced my medication, and normalized my blood sugars. Miraculously, I changed my life and regained my health and well-being.

After I got my health under control, my doctor started referring clients to me, and I was coaching people back to health in my living room. Some would leave the sessions in tears because they were so grateful to have found my program. I became inspired to share what I had learned and to help others end their struggles with sugar and chronic health conditions.

To accomplish my goal, I needed to learn more, so my next step was to attend The Institute of Integrative Nutrition's joint program with Columbia University, where I received my certification as a Health Counselor.

Over the next several years, I also became a trained Meditation Coach, a Dance Fitness Instructor, and an Author of "The Diabetes Coach Approach." I also continued to master cooking techniques to help my clients with food plans, recipes, and meal preparation.

The result was the birth of my company, Great Life Inc., including the development of Sugar-Free Lifestyle Coaching and the creation of programs based upon my signature coaching system: The Sugar-Free Lifestyle Roadmap™, which was designed to teach individuals how to make lasting lifestyle changes and bring their lives back into balance.

A New Beginning

I have come a long way from that young girl who looked forward to the bliss of cookies at the end of her day. Throughout my life, I have experienced hundreds of ups and downs, which began more intensely when I was taken away from my home at an early age.

When I was nine, for reasons unknown to me at the time, my dad showed up at my school, took me out of class, and drove me and my brother to the airport, where we boarded a plane going West. I never got a chance to say goodbye to my mother or siblings, nor did I speak to them during our stay in Nevada.

Several months later, with the help of detectives, my mother found us. As mysteriously as we had left, we returned to Pennsylvania. I was heartbroken when my parents decided not to return to our home and moved us into a series of apartments that they both hated.

Ultimately, my parents split, and my mom died soon after I turned 16. High school became a blur of parties, drugs, and falling in love with my first husband, whom I married three months after school ended.

Despite all the chaos, somehow, I managed to graduate from high school with honors, and while married and raising two young children, I went to college and then to law school. I remained friends with my first husband, but our high school romance did not last. It was not always easy, but we managed to co-parent two young children amidst the turmoil that divorce leaves in its wake. In the late 1980s, I met my current husband, who has stood by my side throughout my compulsion with sugar and my journey to regain my sanity and my health.

Together, we navigated parenting and step-parenting, a bankruptcy that almost brought us to our knees, started new careers, and ultimately, created a life of stability and peace that is full of love, family, friends, and fur babies.

Throughout this journey, I learned that my life experiences, addiction to sugar, the compulsion for certain foods, and the onset of diabetes were all related. This revelation was a lightning bolt that ignited my recovery. I was finally able to stop dieting, change sabotaging behaviors, and learn how to eat in harmony with how my body works to conquer my lifelong cravings.

When I attended The Institute of Integrative Nutrition to become a certified health counselor, I stood up in front of over one thousand attendees and made a commitment to learn why sugar has such a tenacious hold on so many people.

My mission then and now is to create a new way to support the millions of people suffering from the compulsion to consume sugar in all its forms and to empower them to change their relationship with sugar and conquer blood sugar-related health problems.

In the remainder of this book, you will learn how to:

- Eat in harmony with how your body works,
- Identify and eliminate the roadblocks keeping you stuck,
- Develop a strategy to quit sugar and crush cravings.
- Nourish your mind and body with thoughts and foods that lead to vibrant health, and
- Take consistent action to achieve lasting results and enjoy life.

INTRODUCTION:
Why Is Quitting Sugar So Hard?

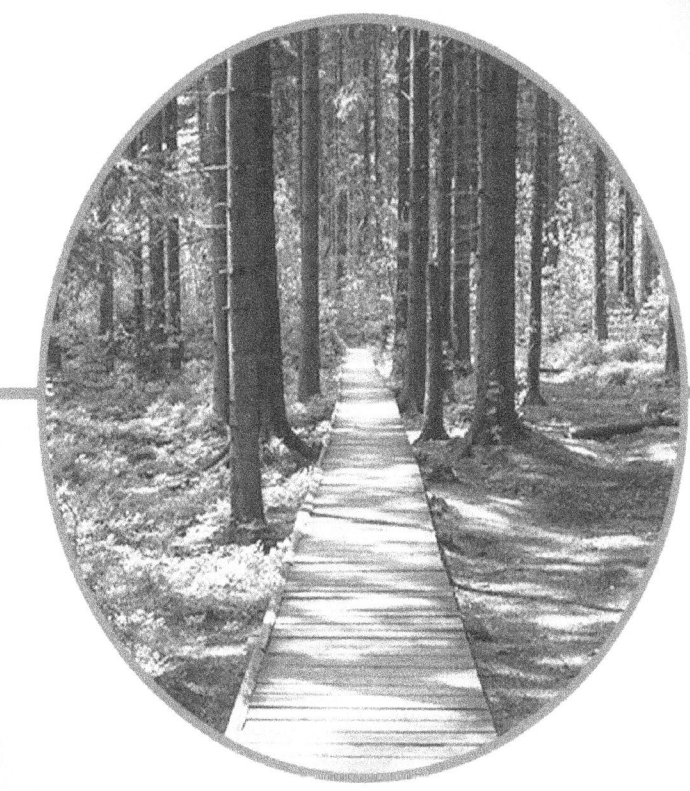

Hiding in the chaos there is calm.

Quiet your mind to hear the silence,

and follow the path to a place of

peace that was there all along.

Janet Sanders

CHAPTER 2
Sugar Consumption Is on the Rise

I am certainly not the only person who has conquered sugar and managed to get their cravings and health under control. There are many people all around the world who have successfully quit sugar, stopped dieting, and manage chronic health conditions. On the other side of the coin, there are thousands (perhaps millions) more who are unable to stop eating sugar and continue to struggle with cravings, yo-yo weight gain, and the onslaught of diseases, such as diabetes, with life-threatening complications.

The wellness movement in the United States has sparked a trillion-dollar industry, and Americans spend more money per capita on health care than any nation in the world. Yet, despite our efforts, sugar consumption, obesity, diabetes, and other chronic illnesses are on the rise.

- An estimated 120 million American adults are either overweight or obese, and at any given time, over 40 million Americans are on some sort of "diet" program.
- In April 2025, the International Diabetes Federation (IDF) reported that the number of adults living with diabetes globally was 589 million, and type 2 diabetes represented approximately 98% of global diabetes diagnoses, although this proportion varies among countries.
- In the United States, in 2021, more than 38 million Americans had diabetes (approximately 90% had type 2 diabetes), and 97.6 million Americans, 18 and older, had pre-diabetes.

Coinciding with the growth of health concerns, the consumption of added sugar is on the rise throughout the globe and is a primary driver of the obesity epidemic. Additionally, the repeated consumption of added sugar increases the roller coaster blood sugar levels that lead to insulin resistance, raising the risk of type 2 diabetes and its complications, including retinopathy, stroke, and both kidney and heart disease.

As it turns out, the reasons so many people consume sugar and other foods that sabotage their health are as complex as the different life experiences that shape our perception of life and how we respond to life's challenges. But there are also some common denominators that shed some light on why it is so hard to change our relationship with sugar.

Sugar is Everywhere

One of the pervasive reasons people consume sugar is that it is everywhere. As a result, it takes some planning and a change of eating habits to avoid it. Many people do not realize that there are many sources of sugar that are digested differently and have varying effects on our bodies.

These sources include:

- Added sugar, which is sugar added to foods during preparation or industrial processing to make them sweet. This includes table sugar, maple syrup, honey, and other sweeteners.
- Naturally occurring sugars such as lactose, which is found in milk and other dairy products, as well as fructose in fruit.
- Hidden sugar refers to foods that don't have sugar in their ingredients but behave like sugar when digested. These foods cause a fast/sharp rise in blood sugar levels along with an elevated insulin response that is similar to the effects of added sugar in our system. Examples include grain-based flour, white rice, and white potatoes.

You will learn more about sugar sources in later sections, including strategies for changing your plate and enjoying alternatives to foods containing various sources of sugar.

Ultra-Processed Foods are Designed to Keep You Hooked

Another more insidious reason that many consume sugar, even when they desperately do not want to, can be traced back to how food is prepared, sold, and marketed. The primary goal of companies participating in the billion-dollar food industry is to get you to eat their food products. It is the job of food company executives to know what people want to eat and to design foods that will make you crave more, even if it threatens your health. They do this by developing what I call "the secret formula." Food companies know that eating a particular combination of fat plus sugar (or fat plus salt, or a combination of all three) will turn on a chemical state in your body that will cause you to want to eat more of that food. These ultra-processed foods are their most profitable, and they create products with these formulas in mind.

Food formulas that encourage compulsive eating, combined with the massive advertising machine and food subsidies that make processed foods a cheap commodity, are truly a recipe for disaster. The result is that millions of people routinely eat highly processed foods with high amounts of sugar, fat, salt, and other synthetic chemicals. I am not suggesting that food industry executives are bad people, but there is no denying that the bulk of our current food industry is based on a system that damages our health and leads to chronic illness.

Processed foods are part of our lives for many reasons. We lead busy, complex lives and turn to processed foods for convenience. We also eat them out of habit, as part of family tradition, and for emotional support.

At this point, some of my clients are ready to run out of the room. But if you are wondering what is left that you CAN eat, don't leave yet. There is no need to give up all family traditions or all prepared foods. As you will learn, my approach offers a balanced way to eliminate added sugar and to choose healthier versions of prepared foods that are free of sugar and contain fewer ingredients that cause you to crave more. This approach is not about deprivation but about making choices that benefit your health and well-being.

Throughout this book, I will teach you how to change your plate in a way that works for your lifestyle and how to eat foods that your tastebuds and body will love. You will learn how to "major" in vegetables, "minor" in healthy proteins of your choice (depending upon whether you are vegan, vegetarian, flexitarian, or carnivorous), and how to choose a variety of "electives" that will help you stay satisfied and on track, such as:

- Bread and other baked goods that do not contain sugar or grain-based flour,
- Healthy fats and oils,
- Substitutes for rice and white potatoes, and
- Low glycemic fruits.

We will also learn about various sugar alternatives, and you will gain clarity about whether sugar alternatives are right for you.

As we will discuss in the next section, a final reason that quitting sugar is challenging is that each of us has a different relationship with sugar. What each of us must avoid differs based on our life experiences, unique biochemistry, and emotional makeup. This means that quitting sugar is not just about the food. You also need to gain clarity about why you are drawn to sugar and develop strategies to let go of habits and behaviors that keep you stuck.

Perhaps the most important thing you can take away from this book is that there are no good or bad foods, including foods containing sugar. The real issue is how a particular food affects you and your body. It does not matter how others feel about that food or how it affects them. Throughout this book, you will learn about the connection between sugar and your mind and body so that you can gain a deep understanding of how sugar, in all its forms, affects both your mental and physical health. When you learn to eat in harmony with how your body works, it makes it easier to stay free from sugar and get back on track when life gets in the way. Remember, this is not about judgment but about discovering what works for you and making informed choices.

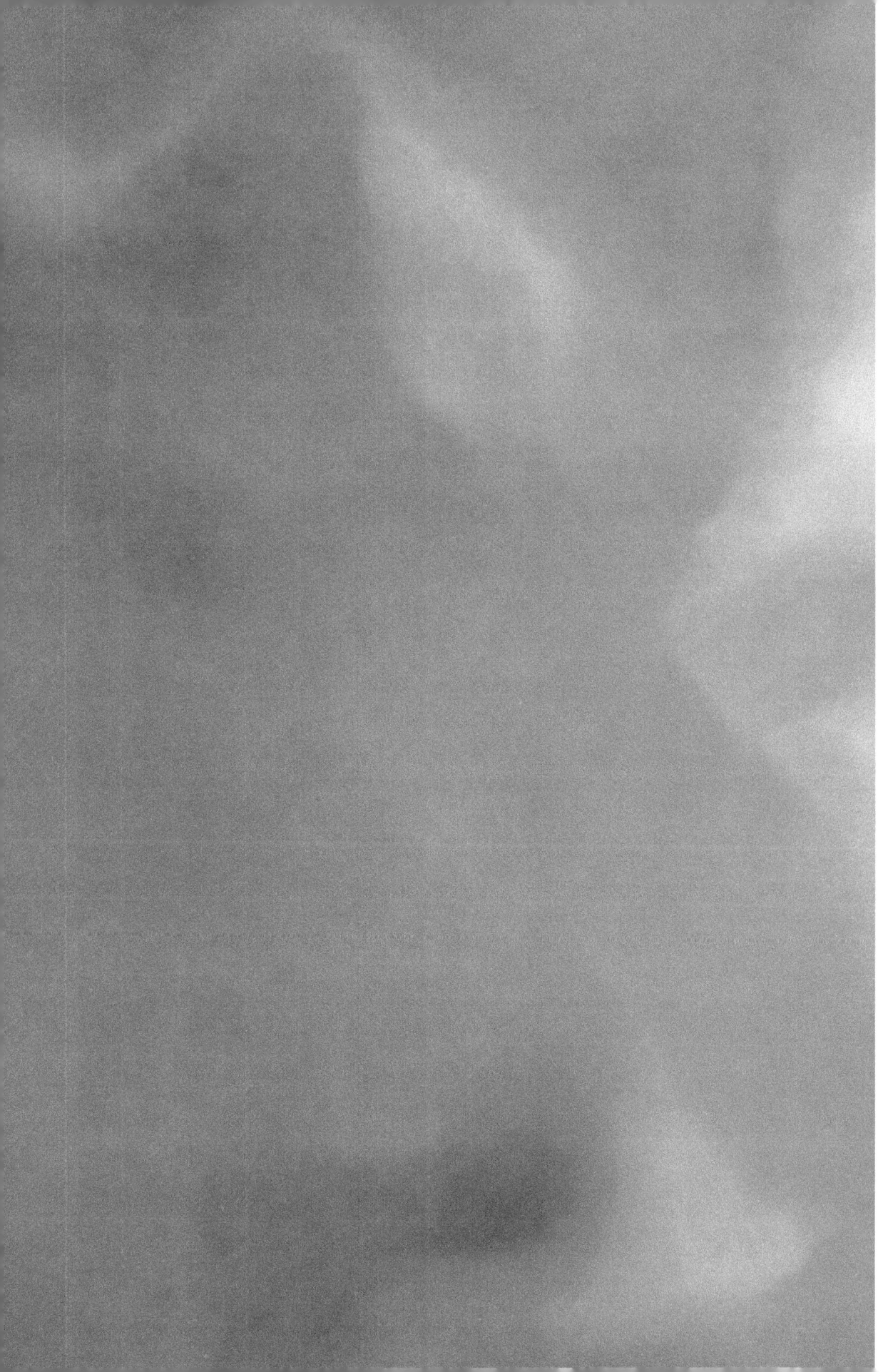

THE SUGAR, MIND, AND BODY CONNECTION

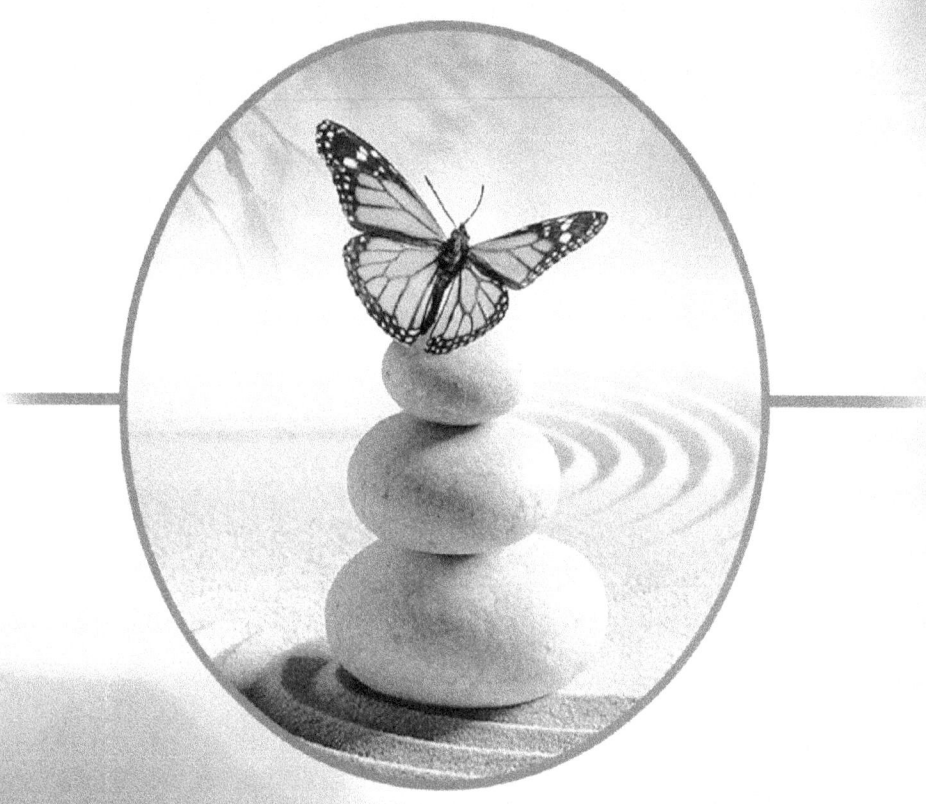

Transform your mind.

Nourish your body.

Change your life.

Janet Sanders

CHAPTER 3
Eating Food Is Enmeshed in Every Aspect of Our Life

Our Brain Is Wired to Enjoy Food

The act of eating food is intricately woven into our physical needs, social habits, reward mechanisms, past experiences, and emotional coping strategies. Most people dislike complexity, and focusing on a diet plan that provides a list of what to eat and what to avoid seems easier at first, until cravings set in. Willpower no longer works, and we are back to eating sugar and other foods that sabotage our health.

I promise that taking some time, in the beginning, to understand why you crave certain foods, what foods are guaranteed to take you off-track, and how to choose foods that are perfect for your physical and emotional makeup will make all the difference. It also helps to stop beating yourself up if you enjoy eating.

A core principle that is at odds with the idea that—if we enjoy eating, we must be doing something wrong—is that our brains are wired to enjoy food as a primal survival mechanism. Your body needs foods that are energy-dense and is drawn to sweet-tasting foods, both because sugar provides a quick energy source and the feeling of pleasure that results from the various chemical reactions that occur in your body when any form of sugar is consumed.

It is not necessary to feel deprived or banish all pleasure from eating. There are a number of strategies to break free from the compulsion to only enjoy foods with sugar in its various forms, including changing your tastebuds to enjoy foods with less or no sugar and eating a variety of energy-dense foods that do not cause the cascade of hormonal reactions that lead to physical cravings. We will explore these and other options as we move through the chapters in this book.

You will also learn a variety of reasons that we are motivated to consume certain foods, including convenience, habit, life situations such as celebrations and family gatherings, physical addiction, and emotional eating, and how to develop strategies to handle these challenges and keep sugar at bay.

The Draw to Sugar Is Both Physical and Psychological

The first step in getting a handle on compulsive eating is to understand that the draw to food can be physical, psychological, or both. Physically, the chemical reactions that occur inside your body when you eat sugar include the release of dopamine in your brain, triggering feelings of pleasure, which, for many, can be addictive, leading to a desire for more sugar to increase these feelings of pleasure.

Additionally, during the digestion process, other hormones, such as insulin, come into play. When you eat foods that cause fast/sharp spikes in both glucose and insulin, this can result in roller-coaster blood sugar levels that lead to sugar cravings and physical addiction to trigger foods that drive physical cravings for either more of the same food or binge eating of other types of food.

For millions of people around the globe, a steady diet of sugar can lead to a condition called insulin resistance that wreaks all sorts of havoc on our system, including:

- Constant cravings for sugar and other carbohydrates,
- Interference with other hormones, such as leptin, which is designed to tell your body when you have eaten enough, and
- Unwanted fat storage and yo-yo weight gain.

In the sections relating to "how your body works," you will learn more about insulin resistance and other hormones that are involved in digestion. In addition to physical cravings, many people have a psychological compulsion and turn to sugar as comfort food in times of stress or emotional upheaval, resulting in an emotional dependence on certain foods.

The bottom line is that we are all prone to the lure of food in varying degrees and for different reasons.

CHAPTER 4
Changing Your Relationship with Sugar

When Quitting Sugar, Your Relationship to Food Matters

If you are prone to the lure of food, are you fighting a losing battle? The answer is no, but to win, you need to have clarity about your personal relationship with food, especially with sugar. There is a big difference between a person who, when faced with certain foods, can simply choose not to consume them and a person who has a physical or emotional compulsion to eat certain foods. The primary difference is the degree to which they are compelled or obsessed with eating certain foods and cannot rely on the mechanisms that occur during the digestion process to signal that they have had enough. Additionally, most who eat compulsively cannot rely on rationality to stop eating, even when they know a particular food is harming them.

Everyone exists somewhere on the continuum between normal eating and addictive or emotional eating.

"Normal" Eating

Most everyone experiences cravings occasionally. The difference is that normal eaters are able to stop and do not experience the compulsion which is the hallmark of addictive or emotional eating.

Physical Cravings or "Addictive" Eating

Characterized by a chemical dependency to trigger foods that drive physical cravings for either more of the same food or that lead to cravings and binging on other foods.

Emotional Eating

Characterized by an emotional dependency to foods that provide comfort and feed a desire to use those foods to cope, self-medicate and/or numb unwanted feelings.

Cravings Trigger Foods

If you crave sweets or other foods, you are not alone. Most everyone experiences cravings at some point, and many may be tempted by sweets and/or choose to overeat in situations such as celebrations or eating out at their favorite restaurant. They may even find themselves overeating in times of stress or seeking comfort from food in troubled times. However, individuals who do not have issues with addictive or emotional eating are able to follow a plan and get back on track, both in the short and long term. We sometimes think of mental willpower as a tool that works for them.

That is why every diet guru can claim their diet works. We all know someone who quit eating sugar or who has successfully lost weight, who can't understand why you can't just get with the program and follow instructions. Likewise, when your doctor or other health provider hands you a food plan, they assume you have been given enough information and good reasons to follow their instructions. For a certain percentage of eaters, this is true.

As you gain clarity about your relationship with food, you may discover that you are one of the lucky ones who can easily stick to a food plan without giving in to sugar. But, for the rest of us who have physical or emotional issues with food, a diet program without a more comprehensive approach does not work. We need a strategy that considers the underlying compulsions and practical strategies for learning how to follow a sugar-free food plan.

Physical Cravings and Addictive Eating Are Common Roadblocks to Quitting Sugar

Physical addiction to one or more foods is characterized by a chemical dependency to trigger foods that drive physical cravings for either more of the same food or lead to cravings and binge eating on other foods. Habits, situations, or emotions can be the initial impetus leading to a trigger food. But once the food is eaten, the physical effect occurs, and the cravings and the obsession with eating more kick in.

Trigger foods act in our bodies in different ways, including:

- causing fast/sharp spikes in both glucose and insulin, resulting in roller-coaster blood sugar levels, with peaks, crashes, and resulting cravings,
- causing cravings due to an engineered combination of sugar, fat, salt, or other highly processed ingredients,
- impacting hormones that regulate appetite (Insulin, Ghrelin, Leptin), leading to increased hunger, inability to stop eating, and
- impacting Neurochemicals that direct our moods and survival functions (Serotonin, Dopamine, and Endorphins), causing imbalances, which can lead to intense food cravings and more desire for trigger foods.

Sugar Sources and Trigger Foods

Sugar and the consumption of trigger foods go hand in hand. The chart below shows the various sources of sugar and provides some insights into how you can begin to put a strategy in place for identifying and eliminating your trigger foods.

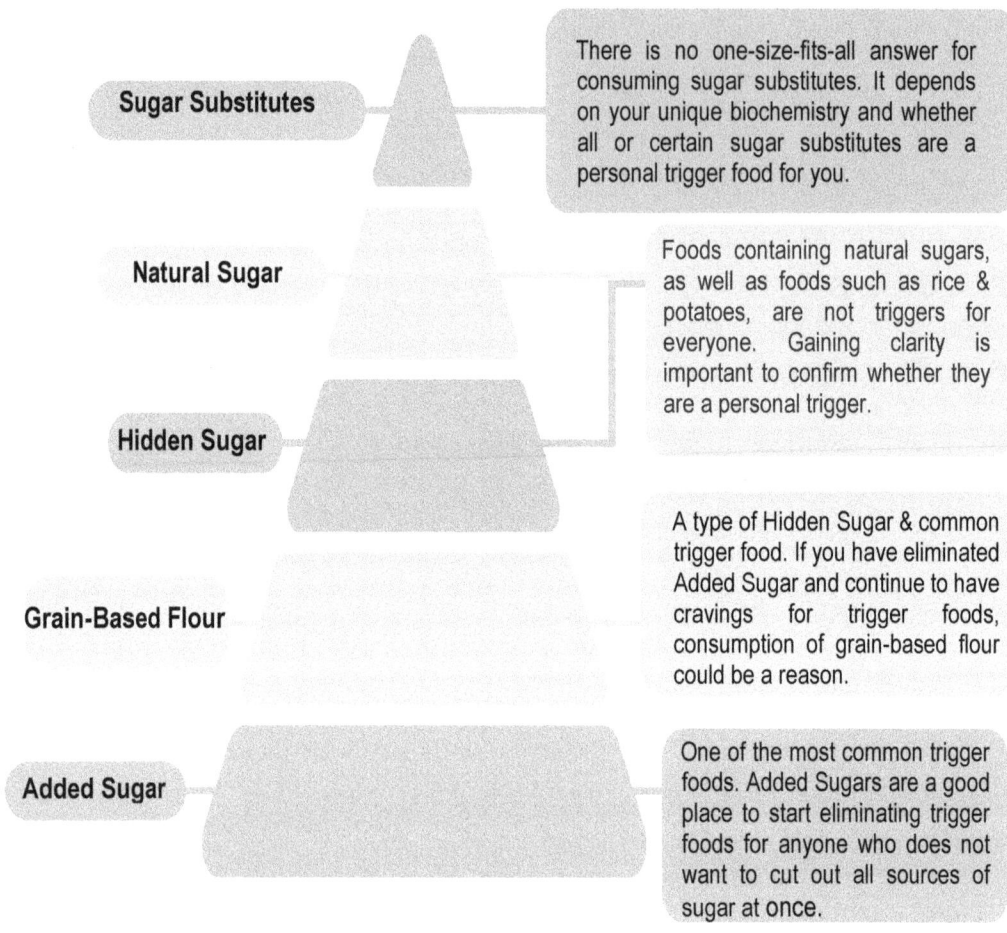

The Relationship Between Trigger Foods and Motivators

There is a difference between a trigger food and the motivation to take that first bite, and it is important to identify both your trigger foods and the motivators in order to eliminate eating trigger foods. Whether food is a trigger that leads to cravings and disordered eating depends on how the food affects your body, based on your unique biochemistry and any other emotional factors.

The chart below provides an overview of Motivators and Related Trigger Foods.

Trigger Food Motivators	Common Trigger Foods
Convenience • Lifestyle factors that lead to a desire for easily available "ultra-processed" foods containing a combination of sugar, salt, and fats that lead to roller-coaster blood sugars and cravings.	Sauces, Marinades, Salad Dressing, Pasta Sauce, Mayonnaise, Nut Butters, Fruit Flavored Yogurt, Soda, Pizza, Pre-made Processed Meals
Sabotaging Learned Behaviors and Habits • Eating certain foods habitually in certain situations, such as watching television, studying for exams, or when feeling bored, leads to ongoing sabotaging behaviors.	**Breakfast:** Cereal, Bagels, Muffins **Lunch:** Sandwiches, Fries, Chips **Dinner:** Potatoes, Rice, Pasta, Pizza **Snacks:** Sweets, Coffee, Cookies, Chips
Life Situations • Eating in reaction to common life situations can lead to disordered eating. Examples include Holidays, Illness, Celebrations, Job Loss, eating at Restaurants, Loss of Family/Friends, or Divorce.	**Sweets:** Chocolate, Cookies, Cake, Ice Cream **Drinks and Snacks**: Coffee Drinks, Bread, Nuts, Potatoes, Rice, Cheese, Chips, Soda
HALT • Letting yourself get too Hungry, Angry, Lonely, or Tired, leading to cravings, eating sugar, or overeating.	**Sweets:** Chocolate, Cookies, Cake, Ice Cream **Drinks and Snacks**: Coffee Drinks, Bread, Nuts, Potatoes, Rice, Cheese, Chips, Soda
Emotional Eating: • Eating to deal with feelings such as Sadness, Anxiety, Stress, Depression, etc.	**Sweets:** Chocolate, Cookies, Cake, Ice Cream **Drinks and Snacks**: Coffee Drinks, Bread, Nuts, Potatoes, Rice, Cheese, Chips, Soda

Emotional Eating Can be a Double Whammy for Those with an Underlying Physical Addiction

For some people, addressing the physically addictive aspects of foods they are drawn to may be all that is needed. But for others, the pull of sugar in all its forms has both a physical and psychological component, and many people turn to food in times of stress or emotional upheaval. Emotional eating is characterized by an emotional dependency on foods that provide comfort and feed a desire to use those foods repeatedly to cope, self-medicate, and/or numb unwanted feelings.

The emotional eater often deals with a double whammy that includes both:

- a need to cope through food, and
- a physical addiction to trigger foods.

Additionally, many emotional eaters suffer from depression and/or anxiety, and they may be reacting to current situations through a lens of past unresolved anger and/or trauma. Emotional eating can also be a desire to recapture happiness through foods associated with past good times or "golden moments" in order to cope with present feelings, such as sadness or anxiety.

Emotional eaters typically do not seek out vegetables or healthy protein to calm their nerves or soothe their souls. Most often, their comfort foods of choice include sugar, bread, cookies, creamy potatoes, chips, and other foods that lead to sugar highs followed by lows, cravings, more food, and, in some instances, a desire for more dopamine --- all leading to a vicious combination of emotional eating and physical dependency on trigger foods.

While the initial bite is pleasurable, the feeling of comfort is usually short-lived, especially hours later or the next day, when guilt and self-loathing over not being able to stop eating set in. The emotional eater is stuck in a vortex of painful eating that often starts with a need to self-medicate, which then leads to eating trigger foods and the ultimate roller coaster ride of sugar highs, followed by the inevitable lows, cravings, more food, and feelings of hopelessness. Every time a person goes on an emotional eating binge, starting over seems harder, and without intervention, their mental and physical health declines.

To conquer emotional eating, individuals must:

- Identify and resolve the underlying emotional issues driving them to food,
- Learn how to cope with feelings without numbing them with food, and
- Eliminate trigger foods that drive the cycle of emotional eating and cravings.

The Good News: You CAN Break Free from Sugar and Experience Vibrant Health

I have been living a sugar-free lifestyle for over 20 years, though I will not say that I never have cravings for my old friend sugar. I have been where many of you are now, and there have been life situations where I have eaten trigger foods and have needed to seek support to get back on track.

I have been an emotional eater with a physical addiction to sugar my entire life. Because of that, I had to learn how to make decisions that led me toward my vision of health rather than away from it. And some days, I still find myself in my pajamas, wrapped in a warm blanket while drinking a cup of tea so that I can keep the sugar monster away and stay centered without reaching for a trigger food that will start the whole mess over again.

In 2001, I began a journey to move from being a frustrated, unhealthy person fighting insulin resistance, diabetes, and depression to someone who found a new beginning by breaking through the barriers keeping me stuck and learning how to enjoy sugar-free, vibrant health. This is the journey that I share in this book, along with a roadmap for how you can do the same.

Although my road to going sugar-free started with a diagnosis of type 2 diabetes, you do not have to be diabetic or even pre-diabetic to experience the same feelings of anxiety and confusion about your health.

In fact, today, there is a whole new term to describe this phenomenon. It's called Diabesity, which describes the physical symptoms that mark the progression from mild insulin resistance to full-blown diabetes.

- Do you find yourself at the mercy of unrelenting food cravings? (particularly for sweets, bread, cookies, etc.)
- Do you experience energy swings that leave you feeling exhausted?

- Do you have stubborn excess pounds, especially around your midsection?
- Have you experienced yo-yo weight gain followed by constant dieting?

If you answered yes to any of these questions, you are in exactly the right place. In the next section, I will share the secrets to successfully going sugar-free and provide an overview of the Sugar-Free Lifestyle Roadmap™, which is the foundation for the remaining chapters of this book. You will learn how to use this book for lasting results, and I will provide coaching tips that will empower you to achieve your desired results every step of the way.

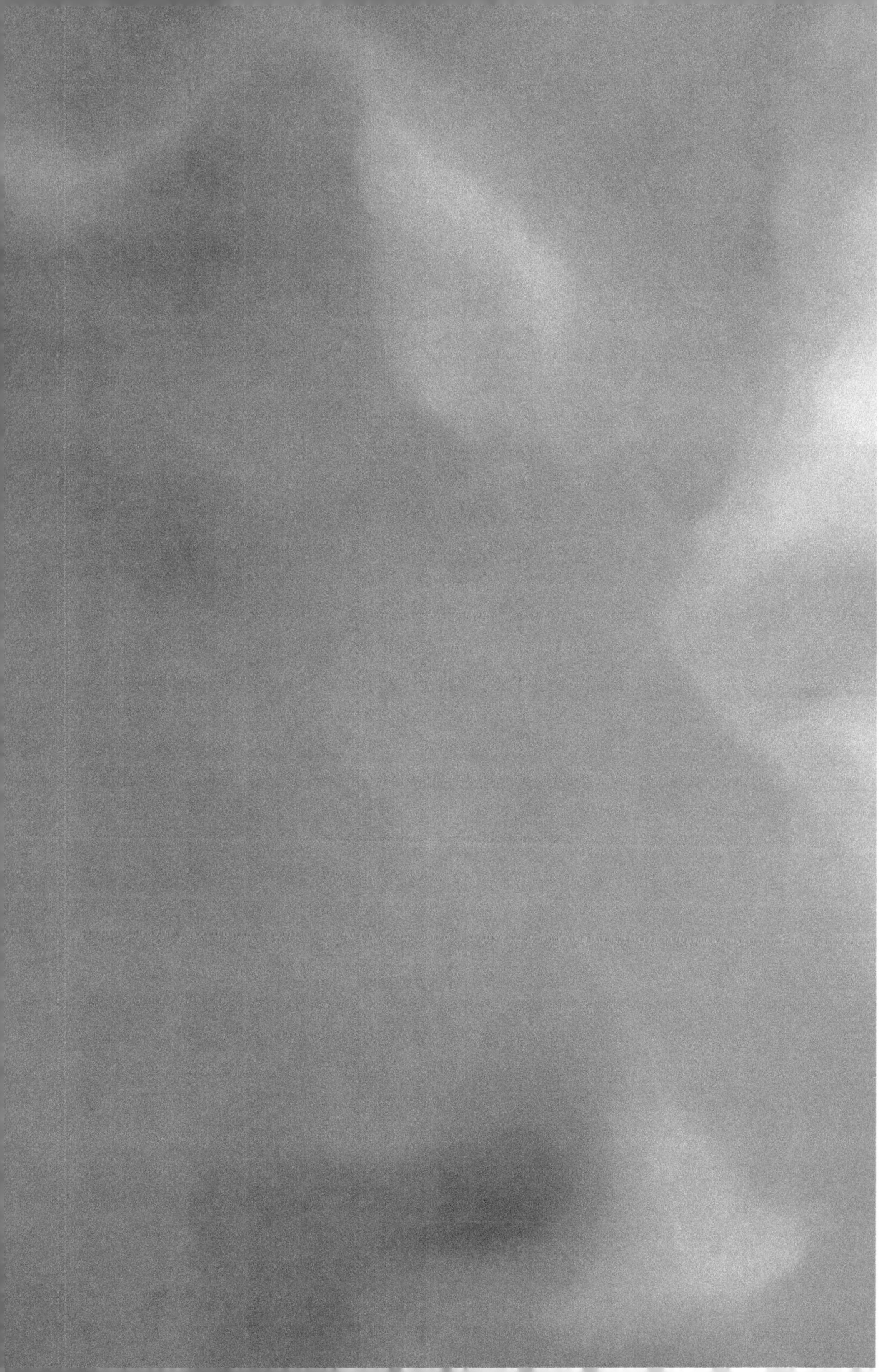

HOW TO USE THIS BOOK TO ACHIEVE RESULTS

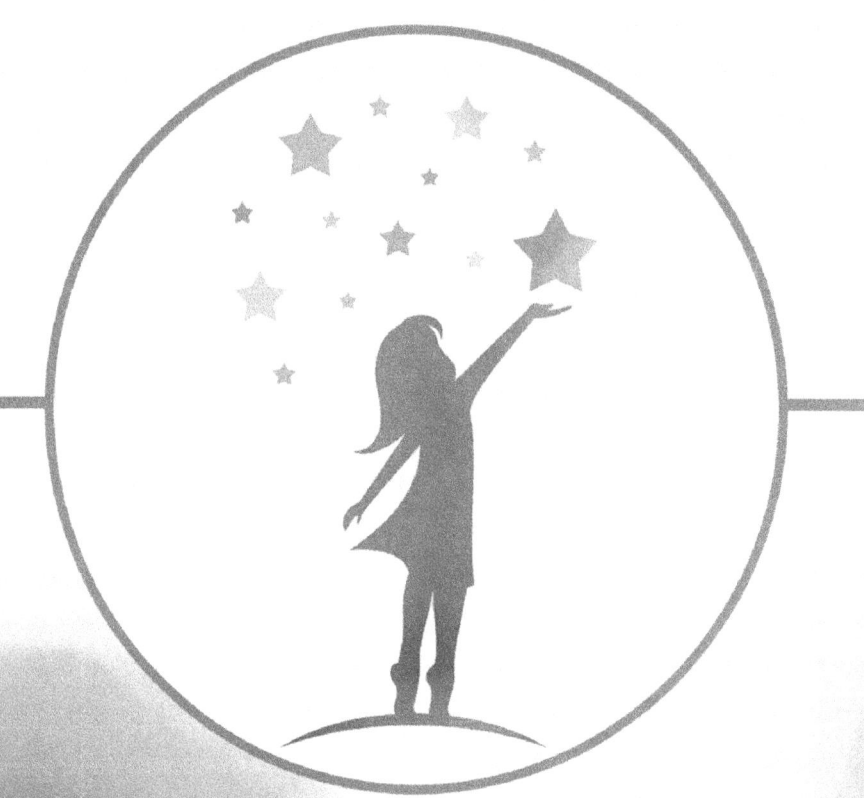

Reach for the stars with your
feet on the ground, carrying
you forward day by day, and
somewhere in the middle, you will
find the life of your dreams.
Janet Sanders

CHAPTER 5
The Roadmap to Sugar-Free Vibrant Health

Breaking Down the Barriers Keeping You Stuck

When I was developing my coaching programs; I started by looking for common denominators shared by individuals struggling with blood sugar health issues. I found that they typically have Roadblocks that sabotage their efforts to quit sugar and improve their health for the long term.

Traditional approaches for quitting sugar or managing blood sugars do not attack the underlying causes of physical food addiction, emotional eating, or roller coaster blood sugars head on. Instead, they tell you to stick with this or that diet, to rely on willpower for results and hope for the best.

As a result, most people, at best, achieve temporary results, but sooner or later, roller-coaster blood sugars return --- cravings and yo-yo weight gain continue, because these roadblocks and underlying causes were never totally eliminated, and new behaviors could not take hold. The most common roadblocks and underlying causes are listed in the diagram below.

The most common roadblocks are set forth in the diagram below.

Roadblocks	Underlying Cause
Resistance to Change	Loss and fear of the unknown
Physical Cravings for Sugar and Other Trigger Foods	• Unaddressed "motivators" to eat sugar and other Trigger Foods • Roller-coaster blood sugars • Body chemistry and natural desire for sweets
Unmanaged Stress & Emotional Eating	• Chronic stress • Learned Behaviors • Life Situations and emotions • Unresolved Trauma

I learned that developing a strategy to clear away the roadblocks and the underlying causes changes everything. Conquering blood sugar health issues in the long term requires a threefold approach:

- Embracing change in order to let go of the past, adapt to new ways of living, and embark on a new beginning
- Learning how to nourish our bodies and make lifestyle changes in all areas, including how we eat, think, and live on a daily basis, and
- Transforming our minds so that we can eliminate the roadblocks keeping us stuck and create an environment that supports lasting change and a life we enjoy.

Putting it All Together with a Roadmap for Success

Once I identified the core components necessary for lasting change, I organized them into a three-phase Sugar-Free Lifestyle Roadmap™. This roadmap serves as the foundation for this book and all my programs. The diagram below provides an overview of the Roadmap and the Steps associated with each Phase.

PHASE ONE: Embrace Change to Break Free from Sugar

- Commit to Making Lasting Changes and Adopting the 4 C's of Change and Resilience
- Connect to Yourself and a Supportive Community to Let Go of the Past
- Consistently Take Action to Quit Sugar and Adapt to a Sugar-Free Lifestyle
- Gain Clarity (Where You Are and Where You Want to Go) to Embark on a New Beginning

PHASE TWO: Nourish Your Body to LIVE Free from Sugar

- Learn How Your Body Works: The Sugar, Mind, and Body Connection
- Implement a Food Plan that Eliminates Personal Trigger Foods
- Validate, Monitor, and Adjust Your Plan
- Enhance Your Food Plan with Exercise, Restful Sleep, and Stress Management

PHASE THREE: Transform Your Mind to STAY Free from Sugar

- Find the Thoughts, Roadblocks, and Eating Patterns Getting in Your Way
- Reverse Sabotaging Thoughts, Habits, and Eating Patterns
- Eliminate Clutter in Your Space to Create an Environment that Supports Lasting Change
- Enjoy Life!

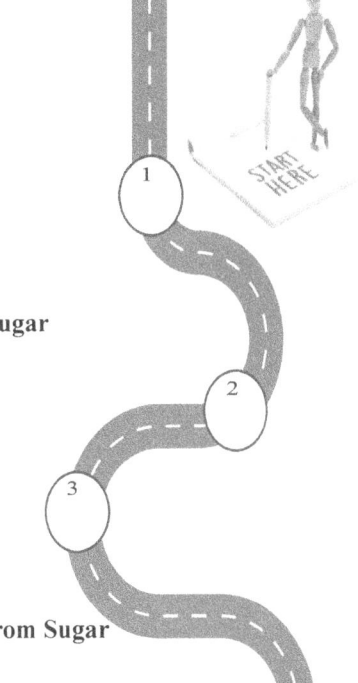

The Roadmap Coaching Format

One of the challenges I grappled with when writing this book was organizing the steps in a way that could accommodate a diverse universe of people who have different health challenges and are at different stages in their health journeys.

Change is not a linear process, no matter where you are or what goals you are trying to achieve. You can't do everything at once, and typically, you find yourself working on one or more goals and priorities at any given time.

To address individual needs, I designed the program to be self-paced, allowing you to adopt the coaching plan gradually and in a way that works for you. The program's 12 steps are organized into 3 phases, and each step is a chapter in this book.

There is no right or wrong way to use this book. You can start at Step #1 and move through the steps sequentially, or choose where you want to start, which steps you want to work on, and the order in which you want to move through the program. My main goal is to provide you with everything you need in an easy-to-follow format, with tips and strategies you can return to whenever you need them. Each Roadmap chapter contains the following sections:

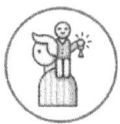

Coach on Your Shoulder

In the section "Coach on Your Shoulder," you'll find personalized coaching guidance tailored for each chapter of this book. Think of me as your dedicated coach, accompanying you every step of the way. My goal is to help you master the concepts presented in each chapter, ensuring you stay on track and continue progressing toward your goals. Together, we will work on developing a sustainable, sugar-free lifestyle, overcoming challenges, and celebrating your successes. With my support, you'll have the tools and motivation to keep moving forward, making lasting changes for a healthier you.

Key Concepts

The "Key Concepts" section is the heart of each chapter, comprehensively explaining the essential topics you'll need to understand and apply. Here, you'll find all the information required to take actionable steps and complete the exercises designed for each chapter. This section is crafted to ensure you grasp the foundational principles and practical insights necessary for your journey. By mastering these key concepts, you'll be well-equipped to implement the changes and strategies outlined, paving the way for your success as you create and maintain your sugar-free lifestyle.

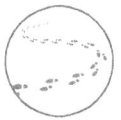

Action Steps

Information alone is not enough; it needs to be combined with action to achieve real progress. In this section, you will find associated tasks and worksheets specifically designed to transform your experience from passive learning to active participation in the creation of your sugar-free lifestyle. By engaging with the tasks and completing the worksheets, you'll move beyond merely understanding the concepts to actively applying them in your daily life. This hands-on approach ensures that you make steady progress, turning knowledge into action and consistently advancing toward your goals.

Takeaways & Highlights

The "Takeaways & Highlights" section provides a concise summary and condensed outline of the key topics covered in each chapter. This section is designed to distill the most essential points, making it easier for you to review and reinforce what you've learned. Having a summary at the end of each chapter allows for quick reference and helps you stay focused on the essential concepts as you move forward. By revisiting these highlights, you can ensure that you have a clear understanding of the material, which will support your continued progress.

Regardless of your approach, the end game is changing your relationship with sugar and achieving your goals. I promise there will be lots of practical tips, guidance, and delicious food to enjoy along the way.

If you need extra support, I have created a coaching community where you can ask questions and connect with me and others who are participating in this journey. The community at www.sugarfreelifestylecoaching.com provides additional resources, including videos, eBooks, daily journals, recipes, and group coaching programs.

CHAPTER 6
Coaching Tips for Success

Eight Ways to Use Coaching Tools to Break Free from Sugar

One of the pervasive myths about changing the way we eat is that all you need is the right information, and combined with willpower, you will get results. Indeed, you can find hundreds of books, articles, and cooking guides that will give you information and tell you WHAT to do in order to conquer sugar and manage blood sugar.

Everyone is aware of the advice to:

- Cut out added sugar,
- Eat vegetables, healthy protein, and fats,
- Exercise more, and
- Reduce stress.

Experts may have slight variations, but I have just given you the basic recipe for living a sugar-free lifestyle, controlling blood sugars, and ending yo-yo weight gain.

If that information is all people need, would there be a pre-diabetes epidemic? Would millions be fighting insulin resistance, obesity, and yo-yo weight gain? The answer is a resounding NO! An important concept to understand is that regardless of changes made, if you go back to your "old" ways, you will find yourself right back where you started or, sometimes, in a worse situation.

In this section, I will share coaching tips and information that support lasting results. The coaching aspect of *Break Free from the Sugar Blues* teaches you HOW to align your behaviors and goals with your vision of health. It adds a new dimension by providing an opportunity to uncover how your thoughts and habits have led you to where you are while providing practical support and guidance to quit sugar and make lasting lifestyle changes.

Below are some suggestions to maximize the benefits of the coaching tools provided throughout the roadmap chapters.

Pick a Good Time to Start: Don't sabotage yourself by starting at a time when you are doomed to failure. On the other hand, no time will be free of all obstacles, so don't depend on finding the PERFECT Time to start. There is no such thing. The important thing is to strike a balance between procrastination and honoring life circumstances that make it difficult to maintain change.

Make a Commitment and Focus on Action, Not Perfection: Commit to what you reasonably think you can accomplish, and take action to meet those commitments. You will be well on your way to cutting back on sugar for better health, even if you don't do every activity perfectly. Remember that what your mind can conceive and believe can be achieved. By giving yourself a new sense of control, even small, consistent changes set the stage for further growth.

Keep an Open Mind: Your mind is like a parachute…it only works when it is open. Many of the concepts will be new to you. If you find yourself particularly resistant to making specific changes, use the tools in the course to discover the source of your resistance.

Take What You Like and Leave the Rest: This program aims to ensure that you have the information, tools, and support you need to make and maintain informed lifestyle decisions. Everyone's biochemistry is different, and there is no perfect way to eat, including sugar and sugar substitutes. Some suggestions will suit you well, and others may not. Ultimately, you will need to develop a plan that fits your needs and lifestyle.

Don't Get Discouraged if You Go Off Track: You have no race or deadline to meet. When faced with a food choice that could lead you away from your goals, ask yourself three questions:

- What are my options?
- What are the benefits and/or consequences of this food choice?

- If I choose to eat this food, what can I do tomorrow to get back on track?

If you stray from your path, the important thing is to get back on track and keep moving forward. When you learn how to bounce back and work on your program at your own pace, you will reap the benefits of this program.

Start a Journal: Writing and recording your thoughts will help you develop your vision, set goals, and master lifestyle success habits. If you don't already have one, purchase a notebook or journal that you can use to enter your thoughts, respond to exercises, and make notes about items you would like to explore further. Not only does journaling help you gain clarity and reduce stress, but it can also help you stay organized by putting all your thoughts, questions, and observations in one place.

Monitor Your Progress: Find a tool you are comfortable with to help you track your daily progress. Recording your blood sugar levels (if you are diabetic), daily food intake, and exercise activities will help you become more aware of your behaviors while keeping you on track as you work towards your goals.

Get Support: If following the program on your own is difficult, one approach is to find a buddy or someone who can provide accountability and support as you progress through the process. Also, be sure to communicate your progress or any issues to your physician and other medical support team members, and reach out to them with questions or when you need medical guidance. You can also find support in our coaching community, where you can ask questions and access various options for connecting with me and others who are participating in this journey with you.

Feeling Stuck? Try Changing Can't to Can

When you feel like you are unable to follow through with ideas or suggestions to incorporate new changes into your daily life, a helpful exercise is to change your inner voice and substitute "I can't" with one of the following:

- I don't want to...
- I am not ready to...
- I am afraid to...
- I would like to, but with some modification(s)

Telling yourself that you "can't" is a way of putting the brakes on and eliminating any possibility of moving forward, but substituting one of the phrases above opens up space to explore why you feel this way and allows the seeds of change to grow.

PHASE ONE:
Embrace Change to Break Free from Sugar

- Commit to Making Lasting Changes and Adopting the 4 C's of Change and Resilience
- Connect to Yourself and a Supportive Community to Let Go of the Past
- Consistently Take Action to Quit Sugar and Adapt to a Sugar-Free Lifestyle
- Gain Clarity (Where You Are and Where You Want to Go) to Embark on a New Beginning

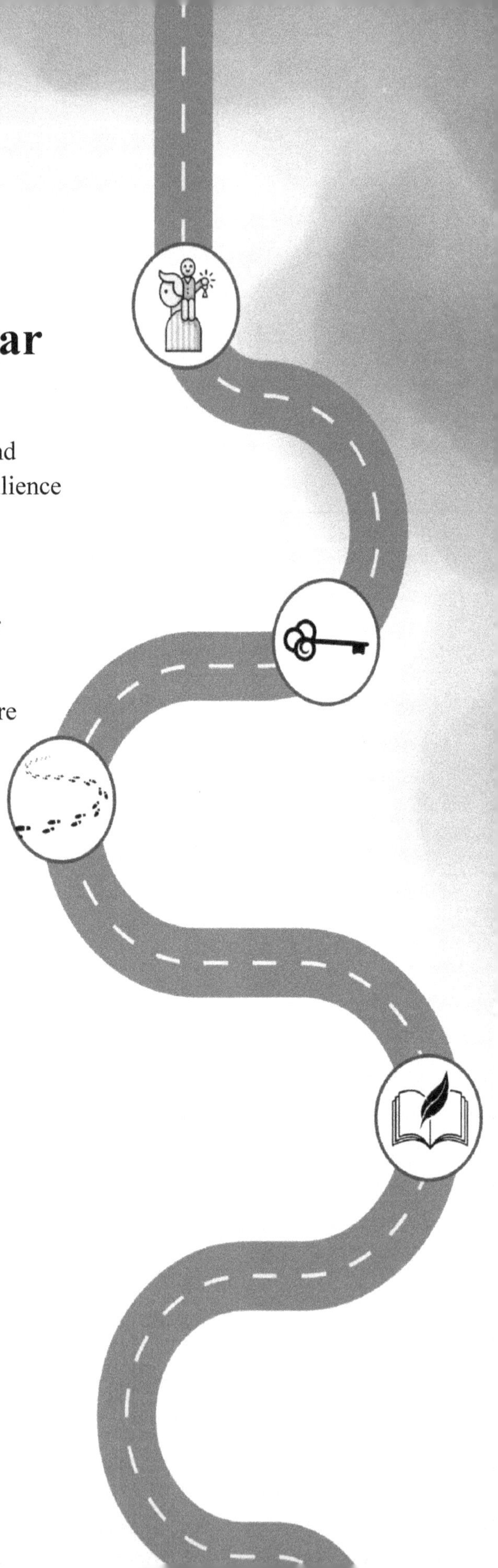

CHAPTER 7
Commit to Making Lasting Changes and Adopting the 4 C's of Change

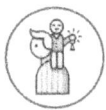

Coach On Your Shoulder

Maintaining a sugar-free lifestyle, conquering roller-coaster blood sugars, and ending yo-yo weight gain starts with managing your mind and learning how to navigate change.

How many times have you wondered why some people seem to easily manage their health while others continue to struggle? I learned the answer is not found in pills or the latest diet plan. Put simply, people who achieve their goals have one thing in common: their commitment to change and to staying resilient in the face of challenges.

Their goals are "must-accomplish goals," not something they might do sometime in the future. The game changer is making a solid commitment to themselves to make necessary changes. This does not mean it is always easy or that they don't have setbacks. But when they stumble, they have a plan to get back on track and are self-motivated to keep moving forward.

In this chapter, you will learn about the power of committing to a plan, which includes embracing four critical elements that I call the 4 C's of Change and Resilience. The Power Quartet — Commitment, Connection, Consistency, and Clarity — is the foundation for meaningful change. Each element is essential to guiding the transformation journey and helping navigate the challenges that arise along the way.

An essential part of committing to change is being ready for it. Although this seems self-evident, many stumble in their efforts to reach their sugar-free health goals because they are not ready to commit to the changes needed to maintain a sugar-free lifestyle. This can lead to feeling like you have failed when all it means is you have some work to do to commit to the process. When you meet yourself where you are, your chances of success increase exponentially because now you know your challenges and roadblocks, and you can put strategies in place to address them rather than beating yourself up and quitting.

Later in this chapter, you will learn about the six stages of change readiness and have the opportunity to complete a Self-Assessment exercise to clarify your priorities and readiness to move through the change process.

Key Concepts

Adopting the he 4 C's of Change and Resilience to Conquer The Sugar Blues

Resilience is a personal superpower you can call on whenever needed. Think of resilience as being like a rubber band. It can stretch and bend but always returns to its original shape. Resilience has one characteristic that makes it even better than a superpower. You don't have to be born with it. When you embrace change, you are also working to make your resilience powers stronger so that you can:

- Overcome obstacles,
- Stay positive when things are difficult, and
- Come back strong after being knocked down.

The good news is that adopting the 4 C's of Change, described below, increases your chances of succeeding in eliminating added sugar, cutting back on other sugar sources, and maintaining a sugar-free lifestyle for the long term.

- **Commitment** fuels drive, motivation, and unwavering dedication to the change you seek. Without genuine commitment, the journey towards transformation can become riddled with doubts and hesitations. True commitment means staying resilient despite obstacles and remaining steadfast in your pursuit regardless of the challenges. Commitment creates a powerful mindset that strengthens resolve, providing the internal motivation and determination required to see the change process through to its completion.
- **Connection** includes an inner connection to self and an outer connection to a supportive community. Both empower you to let go of the past, eliminate sabotaging behaviors, and manifest desired life changes. Internal introspection helps to explore the relationship between thoughts, feelings, and actions, while a community of support—be it family, friends, or a group going through a similar transformation—provides emotional backing, accountability, and a sense of camaraderie.
- **Consistency** is essential for implementing lasting change. Change is a process that results from consistent, repeated actions over time that gradually replace old habits with new ones. Taking small, incremental steps toward identified goals reinforces your commitment and brings you closer to the change you seek. Even small, consistent actions propel you forward, leading to significant changes over time.
- **Clarity** acts as a guiding light on the path to change. Before embarking on any transformational journey, it is crucial to clearly understand where you are (physically and emotionally) and have a vision of what you want to achieve. Clarity enables you to set achievable goals, develop effective strategies, and make informed decisions. It serves as a source of inspiration during challenging times and fuels your determination to stay on course, leading you closer to your goals.

The Six Stages of Change Readiness

Precontemplation: *"I don't see a need for change."*

This is the initial stage where individuals are not yet aware of a problem or the need for change. They may be in denial or unaware of the negative impacts of their current behavior. During this stage, external influences such as information, personal stories, or health scares can help nudge individuals toward recognizing the need for change.

Contemplation: *"I know I should change, and I am thinking about it, but there are still things about the behavior I like---I am not sure I want to change."*

In the contemplation stage, individuals recognize the problem and start considering making a change. However, they may feel conflicted due to the perceived effort, sacrifices, or potential failure associated with the change. The decisional balance here is key—when the perceived benefits of change outweigh the perceived costs.

Preparation: *"I am ready to change, but I don't know how. I need a plan."*

At the preparation stage, individuals are ready to take action and start planning for change. They may take small steps towards the change, like doing research, setting goals, or seeking support. At this stage, the focus is on creating a realistic and achievable action plan.

Action: *"I am ready to change and to take action, although I know there may be challenges and obstacles ahead."*

The action stage involves implementing the change plan. Individuals replace old habits with new ones and make the behavioral changes necessary to achieve their goals. Both repetition of positive behaviors and celebration of achievements during this stage are crucial to maintaining motivation.

Maintenance: *"I am keeping up with my behavior changes, although it is not always easy."*

In the maintenance stage, individuals work to consolidate the gains made during the action stage and prevent relapse. They continue practicing the new behavior until it becomes a habit. This stage often involves developing strategies to cope with potential triggers and sustain the new behavior in the long run.

Relapse: *"I made some decisions that have led me AWAY from my goals."*

Relapse is often considered a stage in the change process rather than a failure. Most people experience setbacks when trying to make a change, which is a natural part of the process. The key is to learn from the relapse, adjust your plan if necessary, and then return to the action or maintenance stage.

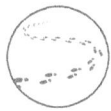

Action Steps

Assess Whether You Are Ready to Quit Sugar

Answer the questions below to determine where you are in the change process. You may not have all the answers at this time. That is OK the questionnaire will help you to see where you might need assistance. Gaining this clarity will enable you to rate your readiness to move forward and create a plan that includes attainable goals rather than trying to take action you are not ready for and setting yourself up for failure.

Precontemplation

- Are you starting to question your sugar consumption habits?
- Do you feel that sugar and related lifestyle habits may be causing negative effects on your health and well-being?
- If yes, what negative effects have you noticed?
- Are you open to learning more about the effects of sugar on your body and mind?

Contemplation

- Have you thought about the benefits of reducing or eliminating sugar and how it could improve your life?
- What are some of the pros/benefits of reducing or eliminating sugar?

- What are some of the cons or things that you are anxious about when it comes to reducing or eliminating sugar?
- Do you find yourself thinking about making changes in your sugar consumption and related lifestyle habits within the foreseeable future?

Preparation

- Have you set a clear intention to live a sugar-free lifestyle? If no, what is standing in your way?
- Have you started to research how to successfully reduce or eliminate sugar?
- Have you established specific/achievable goals for reducing your sugar intake? If no, do you need assistance? If yes, what are the top 3 goals you have identified?
- Have you started to create an action plan? (Do not worry if your action plan is incomplete; you will have an opportunity to develop a detailed action plan in future steps.)
- Have you made plans to deal with situations or triggers that may tempt you to consume sugar? If yes, what are some triggers you have identified?
- Are you ready to take concrete action within the next month? If no, what stands in your way, and when will you be ready to take action?

Action

- Have you started implementing changes in your diet and related lifestyle habits to reduce your sugar intake? If yes, what are some changes you have implemented?
- Are you eliminating added sugar?
- Are you cutting back on natural sugars?
- Are you avoiding "hidden sugar" such as grain-based flour, rice, and white potatoes?
- Do you need help refining your food plan?
- Are you actively practicing behaviors that help you stay away from sugar? If yes, what are some of the behaviors that are helping?

Maintenance

- Have you successfully avoided or minimized sugar consumption for a sustained period? If not, proceed to the Relapse section and answer those questions.
- Do you feel confident in your ability to maintain a sugar-free or low-sugar lifestyle? If no, what are some of the obstacles in your way?
- Are you actively reinforcing positive habits and strategies to stay on track in the face of temptations or difficult situations? If yes, what are some of those habits/strategies?

Relapse

- Have you experienced any instances of consuming added sugar after starting the process of eliminating added sugar? If yes, has this been a limited experience or multiple occurrences?
- Have you experienced any instances of consuming other sources of sugar that you planned to eliminate or reduce, that you consider a setback? If yes, has this been a limited experience or multiple occurrences?
- Do you view relapse as a learning experience rather than failure?
- If you feel you are "failing," where do you think those thoughts come from, and how do those thoughts affect you?
- If you had a setback with added sugar or other sources of sugar, were you able to identify what led to it and learn from the experience?
- If you have experienced a setback, have you identified some steps you can take to get back on track? If yes, what are those steps?
- Do you need help to stop eating sugar? If yes, have you sought support from a group or professional?
- Are you prepared to recommit to your goals if you encounter setbacks and to take action to get back on track?

Complete the Change Readiness Rating

Based on your answers in the Change Assessment, rate yourself using the chart below to confirm where you are and where to focus your efforts. If you are having issues staying on track, both the assessment and rating below may offer some clues.

For example, you might agree that you are ready to take action, but still find things about eating sugar you like, which can lead to confusing and conflicting behaviors. Most people have conflicting feelings when it comes to making any change. By looking honestly at where you are, you can start to address underlying issues and move forward with more clarity.

How often do you agree with each statement below?	Never	Rarely	Sometimes	Always
Pre-Contemplation. "I don't see a need for change in my relationship with sugar."				
Contemplation. "I know I should change, and I am thinking about it, but there are things about sugar I like. I am not sure what I want to change."				
Preparation. "I am ready to change & adopt a sugar-free lifestyle, but I don't know how to move forward. I need a plan."				
Action. "I am ready to change and take action, although I know challenges may be ahead."				
Maintenance. "I am keeping up with my behavior changes, although it is not always easy."				
Relapse. "I make some decisions that lead me away from my goals. I need to reflect, adjust, and take action to get back on track."				

Takeaways & Highlights

Resilience is a set of learn behaviors that help you to:

- Overcome obstacles,
- Stay positive when things are difficult, and
- Come back strong after being knocked down.

The 4 C's of Change, which include Commitment, Connection, Consistency, and Clarity, increase your chances of succeeding in eliminating added sugar, cutting back on other sugar sources, and maintaining a sugar-free lifestyle for the long term.

The six stages of change readiness include;

- **Precontemplation**. "*I don't see a need for change.*"
- **Contemplation**. "*I know I should change, and I am thinking about it, but there are still things about the behavior I like---I am not sure I want to change.*"
- **Preparation**. "*I am ready to change, but I don't know how. I need a plan.*"
- **Action**. "*I am ready to change and to take action, although I know there may be challenges and obstacles ahead.*"
- **Maintenance**. "*I am keeping up with my behavior changes, although it is not always easy.*"
- **Relapse**. "*I made some decisions that have led me AWAY from my goals.*"

Tips for navigating the change process:

- **Determine Your Readiness for Change**. Assess whether you are genuinely motivated to change or are driven by external pressures. Authentic change stems from a deep, personal desire for growth.
- **Identify Goals**. Clearly defining your goals will guide your path and help you stay focused.
- **Accept Imperfection**. Acknowledge that change is not always smooth and may involve setbacks. Embrace imperfections as opportunities to learn and grow.
- **Be Willing to Step Out of Your Comfort Zone**. Change often requires leaving familiar territories and venturing into the unknown. Are you willing to take calculated risks and embrace uncertainty?
- **Find a Support System**. Take steps to establish a supportive network of family, friends, or mentors who can offer encouragement during challenging times.
- **Develop Self-Compassion**. Change may involve facing past mistakes or confronting personal weaknesses. Treat yourself with kindness and understanding.

- **Persevere Through Challenging Times.** Stay committed to the process, even when obstacles arise. True transformation may take time, dedication, and patience.
- **Stay Open to New Ideas and Perspectives.** Willingness to learn and adapt facilitates smoother transitions.
- **Celebrate Progress.** Acknowledge and celebrate even the smallest steps forward. Positive reinforcement reinforces your commitment to change.
- **Visualize Success.** Picture yourself succeeding in your transformed state. Visualization can strengthen your determination and help you maintain focus on your ultimate goal.

CHAPTER 8
Connect to Yourself and a Supportive Community to Let Go of the Past

Coach on Your Shoulder

Regardless of why you choose to eliminate or cut back on sugar, living a sugar-free lifestyle is a profound change. Sometimes, this change is a welcome challenge. Often, it is thrust upon you for health reasons. Regardless of how the change occurs, the change process involves three distinct phases: Letting Go, Adapting, and New Beginnings. Many people get frustrated with this concept. A common reaction is, "I don't want to think about how change works; I just want to change my diet and move on." However, each phase is integral to successful transformation, and when the process is ignored, it often ends in frustration and an inability to stay on track.

In this chapter, you will learn the importance of Letting Go for moving forward and why the process of letting go is aided by the connection both to self and to a supportive community. The "Letting Go" Exercise at the end of the chapter will help you to identify the things standing in your way of letting go of the past and to take the next steps to create your community of support.

Key Concepts

The Three Phases of Change: A Journey of Transformation

The three phases of change are sequential milestones on the journey of transformation.

- **Letting go** allows for the release of old patterns and involves relinquishing old habits, beliefs, or ways of doing things. It is essentially acknowledging the end of what was and creating the space for a fresh start, unburdened by past limitations.
- **Adapting** is a transitional period where you are between the old and the new. It is a time of opportunity as you acquire new skills, explore various strategies, and discover ways to move forward.
- **New Beginnings** mark the realization of positive change. This phase provides closure and a sense of achievement. You start to feel comfortable with your new reality, establishing new routines and habits, and preparing for future transformations.

Each phase in the change process equips you with the tools and mindset to turn change from a daunting challenge into a platform for growth and revitalization. In this chapter, we will delve more deeply into the first phase, "Letting Go," and explore how nurturing a connection to yourself and becoming part of a supportive community are indispensable elements for letting go and changing your long-term relationship with sugar.

The Dynamics of Letting Go of the Past

Inherent in every change is an ending. When faced with a changing situation, our reactions range from denying, ignoring, or embracing the fact that an ending has occurred. Often overlooked, an empowering aspect of change is letting go of the past.

If you can embrace the ending, you can create the space to create a new beginning, which is one of the great secrets of change. Letting go is a form of mental and emotional decluttering that involves relinquishing old habits, beliefs, or ways of doing things. It's about acknowledging that the current state may no longer be relevant or effective. It essentially ends what was and creates the space for what might be

Unfortunately, letting go is incredibly difficult for most people because it requires accepting that the status quo is no longer sustainable or suitable. In many instances, anger at having to make a change and fear of living without things that helped us get through the day hold people back from making a beneficial change. It could be something as simple as waking up ½ hour early to fit in a morning walk or choosing not to eat a huge plate of French fries when you go out to lunch on Saturday afternoon.

When I was diagnosed with type 2 Diabetes, I realized that the old me (the one who ate chocolate chip cookies to soothe my nerves and worked late into the night, fueling myself with carbohydrates) had to give way to something new. At first, the realization was scary. My ability to use sugar as a crutch was ending. What was I going to do now? I was so accustomed to abusing my body and eating my way through situations that I wasn't sure how I would handle anything in my life.

If I wanted to stop repeating the same patterns and move forward, I would have to stop resisting the new and holding onto the obsolete. By shedding outdated patterns and beliefs, I have finally learned how to create space for new perspectives and approaches to challenges. Letting go is like clearing the canvas before painting a new picture, allowing for a fresh start unburdened by past limitations.

The Importance of Connection

There are two essential elements involved in transformative connections:

As we have been discussing, the first step is fostering a deep connection to oneself, so that you can get in touch with the emotions and behaviors that are getting in the way of making necessary changes. The second is developing a connection to a supportive community, including your healthcare team.

Making the transition to a sugar-free lifestyle can be isolating at times, but you don't have to go through it alone. Support from a community or other resources can offer encouragement, advice, and a sense of belonging. They can also hold you accountable, celebrate your victories, and help you bounce back from setbacks.

Those who are most successful with change seek many different forms of support. The diagram below lists the types of professionals or support groups you might enlist to help you reach your goals.

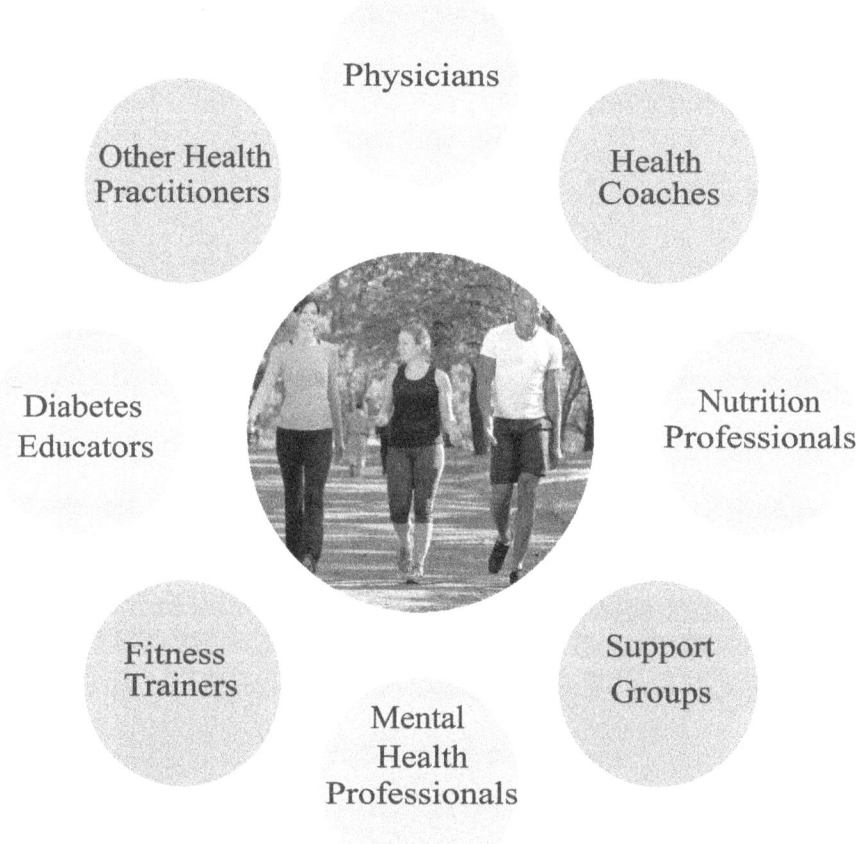

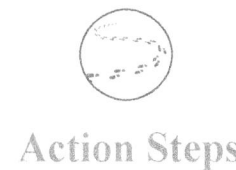

Action Steps

Complete the Changing Your Relationship to Sugar Exercise

This exercise aims to assess your current relationship with sugar and identify your feelings about making a change. As you answer the questions below, you will uncover any feelings and habits rooted in the past that might be getting in the way of letting go of the past, quitting sugar, and adopting new behaviors.

What is Ending if You Let Go of Sugar?

What will change as you let go of your sugar consumption? This might include daily habits, certain foods, or emotional connections. Write down a list of these things. Some examples that might apply to you:

- Eating sugary desserts after dinner
- Grabbing sugary snacks during work breaks
- Using sugary treats as a reward or comfort
- Celebrating with cake and cookies
- Emotional eating with sugary foods when stressed or upset

What Did You Enjoy About the Things You Need to Let Go Of?

What were some of the positive aspects of the sugar-related activities listed above? What did you gain or enjoy from eating sugar, even if it was temporary? For example, eating sugar during work breaks might have been a means of escaping boredom. Eating when stressed can ease feelings of stress or anxiety without having to face these feelings or make an effort to start new habits, such as meditating or taking a walk.

- I enjoyed the taste of these foods
- The candy bar gave me a quick energy boost
- Celebrations felt special with a sweet dessert
- Sugary foods provided comfort and offered an escape from stress.

How Do You Feel About Quitting Sugar and the Changes You Will be Making?

It is natural to have feelings about letting go of foods and experiences that, up until now, have been a big part of your life. Recognizing and understanding these feelings is essential in accepting and moving forward. You may have mixed feelings or resistance, such as feeling a combination of excitement about positive health changes along with nervousness or fear about how you will handle cravings or get through tough times without sugar. Here are some questions to guide you.

- What emotions come up as you think about letting go of sugar?
- Are there any fears or apprehensions associated with these changes?
- Do you feel a sense of loss associated with a specific change?
- Are any of your habits surrounding sugar founded in family traditions?
- What positive feelings or hopes do you have about these changes?

What Foods or Activities Can Help You Let Go of Sugar?

The final step in the letting-go process is finding replacements for sugar and related activities. Whether it's a food or an activity that you want to change, identify what you enjoyed about it or what it fulfills. Suppose you can figure out what a food or activity represents to you. In that case, you can find another food or a non-food activity that provides similar benefits without relying on sugar. In some instances, you might discover that it was something you don't enjoy but do out of habit or because it satisfies an underlying need relating to events or relationships from your past.

Everyone is different, and there are no right or wrong answers to why sugar has a hold on you. The key is understanding why you need sugar and identifying something you can put in its place that will fit the needs of the new you.

If you find yourself stuck and unable to move forward with your Sugar-Free Lifestyle Program, here is another short exercise that can help you let go of foods or activities so that you can move forward with a renewed sense of peace about the changes you are making. Fill in the blanks for each statement below.

- Before I decided to practice a sugar-free lifestyle, I enjoyed the following:
- The things I like best about (doing this activity/eating this food) are:

- Giving up this food/activity or making a change makes me feel:
- A food/activity that I can put in its place is:

Sample Responses:

- Before I decided to practice a sugar-free lifestyle, I enjoyed relaxing at the coffee shop with a sugar-laden "designer" coffee drink and pastry.
- The thing I like best about (doing this activity/eating this food) is the atmosphere and hanging out with a friend.
- Giving up this food/activity or making a change makes me feel both sad and angry that I can't do what I want.
- A food/activity that I can put in its place is enjoying a cup of tea and a healthy snack at home with a friend, or I can go to a coffee shop, choose a sugar-free beverage, and bring my own snack.

Takeaways & Highlights

The three phases of change include Letting Go, Adapting, and New Beginnings.

- The phases of change are sequential milestones on the journey of transformation.
- Letting Go allows for the release of old patterns,
- Adapting enables the development of new skills, and
- New Beginnings mark the realization of positive change.

Tips for moving through the 3 phases of change:

- **Connect to Yourself**. Being connected to yourself fosters self-compassion and self-acceptance, which are essential for overcoming setbacks and staying resilient during the change process. Taking care of yourself and practicing self-compassion sets the stage for letting go of the past and making time for activities that nourish your body and mind. Remember to be kind and understanding towards yourself when you face challenges or setbacks.

- **Let Go of the Past**. Inherent in every change is an ending. When faced with change, our reactions run the gamut from denying, ignoring, or embracing the fact that an ending has occurred. Letting go of the past is an empowering aspect of change. If you accept the ending, you can create the space to embrace a new beginning, one of the most potent secrets of change.
- **Connect to a Community of Support**. Human beings are inherently social creatures, and having a supportive community can significantly impact the success of your transformational journey. There are many ways to gain support from professionals and peers. Both can help you learn how to adapt to a sugar-free lifestyle while providing valuable insights, accountability, and encouragement along the way.

If you still find that you are stuck:

- Find a support person you can talk to and brainstorm with to get clear about what is holding you back and how you might be able to address your feelings.
- Examine some of the significant changes/transition periods in your life. How did you react then? When change comes, do you tend to ignore, deny, or embrace endings?

CHAPTER 9
Consistently Take Action to Quit Sugar and Adapt to a Sugar-Free Lifestyle

Coach on Your Shoulder

A well-known children's riddle asks: "How do You Eat An Elephant?" ANSWER: "One bite at a time." That sums up the period of Adapting, which is the bridge between the old and the new, where you give yourself the time and space to start taking action, learn from your experiences, and build resilience.

Without this phase, the change to a sugar-free lifestyle would be abrupt and potentially overwhelming. Adapting tames the overwhelm by letting you take small, consistent steps so that you can move forward a little bit at a time while gaining knowledge and confidence.

For many people, this can be an incredibly frustrating time where you are stuck between the old and the new, and although you know you can't go back to your old ways, you are not 100% sure of how to move forward. This is a time when you might need to "fake it until you make it." Even if you are scared or unsure of the perfect way to conquer sugar, taking consistent action will give you the confidence to follow through in Phase 2, where you will eliminate trigger foods and create a Food Plan that works for you. In this chapter, you are going to learn how to:

- Navigate through the Adaption Phase of your sugar-free lifestyle
- Identify sugar sources and types of carbohydrates
- Start your new way of eating by finding and replacing added sugar

Eight Action Steps to Help You Find and Replace Added Sugar

- Read labels to find added sugar.
- Stop adding sugar to food, recipes, and beverages.
- Learn about alternative sweeteners.
- Eliminate soda (including diet).
- Replace salad dressings that contain added sugar.
- Replace yogurt containing added sugar with plain yogurt (and flavor the yogurt yourself.
- Replace high-sugar smoothies with no added sugar or low-natural-sugar alternatives.
- Replace pantry items (such as condiments, canned goods, and prepared foods) with brands containing no added sugar.

This may be totally new for some of you and a refresher for others. Although following a certain order when engaging in these activities is not required, I recommend starting with "Find Added Sugar" and "Stop Adding Sugar to Food, Recipes, and Beverages." These two steps are critical whether you are just starting or beginning again after a period of relapse. You can't do everything at once, and the activities are organized in a way that lets you explore them in an order and at a pace that works for you. Details and guidance for the eight action steps are in the Action Steps section of this chapter.

Keep moving forward, establishing new habits, and using this chapter as an anchor to guide you through the process of eliminating added sugar and the roller-coaster blood sugars and cravings that accompany it. Ultimately, in Phase 2, you will build upon eliminating added sugar by eliminating sources of hidden sugar and cutting back on natural sugar.

Cold Turkey or Gradual Changes?

If you are unsure which approach to take, here are some questions to help you decide whether to start slowly or quit added sugar more quickly.

- What is your tolerance for drastic change? If you find yourself overwhelmed trying to do too much all at once, try cutting out added sugar gradually.

- Do you have a health condition that requires you to cut added sugar all at once? If the answer is yes and it is difficult, get support to go cold turkey.
- Is added sugar a trigger food for you? If you are likely to binge or keep eating it (even if you only have a small amount), it is best to quit all at once.
- Did you start slowly but find that you are not achieving the results you were looking for? If yes, you might need to rethink your approach and just dive in.

Some days may not be "perfect," but you can pat yourself on the back for making daily decisions that will move you toward your vision of health. Use this time as an opportunity to try new things and to let go of any negative self-talk as you follow along.

In Phase 2, we will delve deeper into creating a Food Plan that eliminates all added sugar and cuts back on natural and hidden sugars. You will also learn how to eliminate personal trigger foods and how to add foods that enhance your sugar-free lifestyle.

Key Concepts

The Complex Relationship Between Sugar and Carbohydrates

In order to eliminate added sugar and cut back on other forms of sugar, you need to know where to find it. And to find it, you need to know what sugar is, so let's start there. The first thing to know is that every food you eat is made up of 3 very important components:

- **Macronutrients**. These are the building blocks of the foods we eat. Every food contains some combination of protein, carbohydrate, and fat. (A food does not have to include all 3, but every food contains one or two of these macronutrients.)
- **Micronutrients**. The term micronutrients refer to vitamins and minerals that are vital to the healthy development of your body, disease prevention, and well-being.

- **Phytochemicals**. The nutrients from plant foods that enhance health and fight disease are called Phytochemicals.

Macronutrients, and more specifically, carbohydrates, play a significant role in the sugar equation. No food category is as widely discussed or misunderstood as carbohydrates, a primary energy source for your body.

Carbohydrates have by far the most significant impact on blood sugar levels (which in turn affect insulin production, fat storage, and fat burning). Controlling both the quality and quantity of carbohydrates you eat will ultimately produce the best blood sugar results.

You are not going to avoid all carbohydrates. Remember the following guiding principle when selecting carbohydrates, and you will rarely go wrong. The longer your body has to wrestle with a carbohydrate to break it down into glucose, the slower the rise in glucose in your blood. You want to strive to include good-quality complex carbohydrates in your food plan that do not contribute to dramatic swings in your blood sugar levels and subsequent spiked insulin responses.

Four Categories of Carbohydrates

It might surprise you to know that carbohydrates are not food at all but are a collection of molecules consisting of carbon, oxygen, and hydrogen. A single carbohydrate molecule is called a "saccharide," a fancy word for a sugar molecule.

Carbohydrates are classified into several different types based on the number of sugar molecules they contain, and each type metabolizes in our body differently. How these molecules are arranged is at the heart of the great mystery of sugar and the many reasons it has such an enormous effect on your mind, body, and overall health.

Below is an introduction to the four types of carbohydrates.

- **Monosaccharides** are the simplest form of carbohydrates and are the only form that can be directly used by our cells for energy. During digestion, every carbohydrate food you eat is ultimately broken down into one or more of the simple sugars Glucose, Fructose, or Galactose.

- **Disaccharides** are made up of two sugar units that are broken down into their constituent components during the digestion process. Examples are sucrose (commonly known as table sugar), lactose (found in dairy), and maltose.
- **Oligosaccharides** are a type of complex carbohydrate composed of 3 to 10 simple sugar units. They play various roles, including functioning as prebiotics (substances that feed beneficial gut bacteria). They are found in beans, whole grains, broccoli, cabbage, and other vegetables.
- **Polysaccharides** are complex carbohydrates made up of more than ten simple sugar units and sometimes up to thousands. Vegetables, fruit, grains, and beans are all complex carbohydrates.

All Disaccharides, Oligosaccharides, and Polysaccharides are ultimately broken down into Monosaccharide sugar units (Glucose, Fructose, Galactose) during the digestion process.

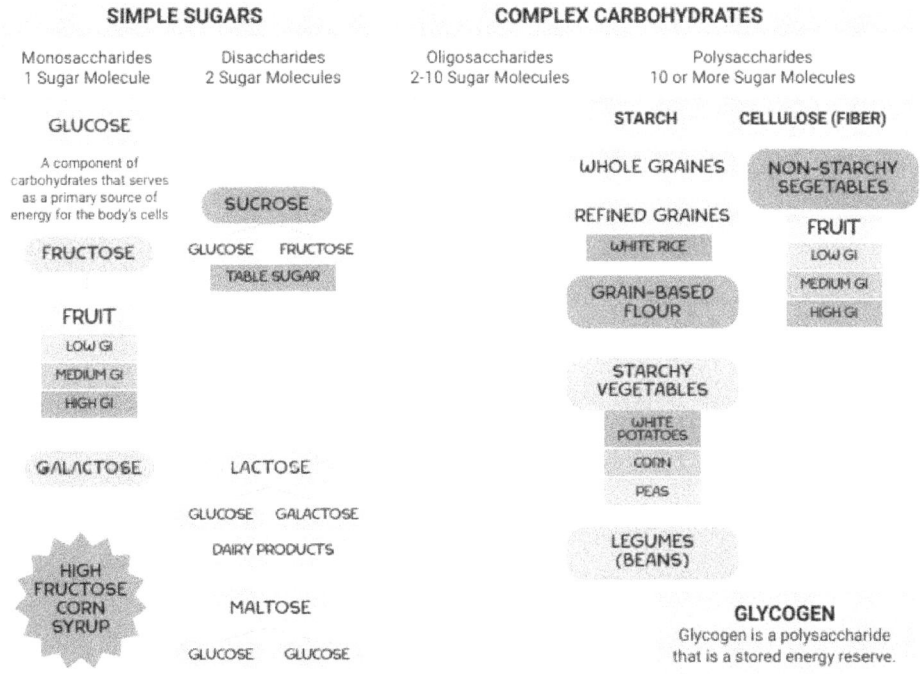

Not All Carbohydrates Are Created Equal

When carbohydrates are metabolized during the digestion process, a portion will be broken down into sugar and will enter our bloodstream to be used by our cells for energy or transported to our liver to be stored for later energy use --- or some might be stored as fat. Even whole grains are a type of starch that will ultimately break down into sugar, so I classify them as a source of hidden sugar. The endosperm of a whole grain, which is the part that contains energy, is mainly made up of starches. The bran and germ of the grain are also part of the whole grain, and the germ contains many vitamins and minerals.

Not all carbohydrates are processed in the same way. The amount of carbohydrates consumed and the rate at which the processed sugar enters our bloodstream profoundly affect blood sugar levels, cravings, and how fat is stored in our bodies. Rapid absorption can lead to swift spikes in blood sugar levels accompanied by a sharp rise in insulin, especially if consumed in large quantities or without other macronutrients like fiber, protein, or fat.

How fast the sugar enters your bloodstream, triggering various physical reactions, depends on several factors, including the type of carbohydrate, how the food was processed, the mix of fiber, fat, and protein, and the food's physical form.

Type of Carbohydrate

Carbohydrates consisting of either one or two sugar molecules have a small structure, which allows them to be quickly absorbed and used by the body. This rapid absorption can lead to swift spikes in blood sugar levels accompanied by a sharp rise in insulin, especially if consumed in large quantities or without other macronutrients like fiber, protein, or fat.

Complex Carbohydrates, including Whole Grains and Non-Starchy Vegetables, generally take longer to digest, resulting in a more gradual increase in blood sugar levels. This is due to a combination of their low sugar content, along with a more complex molecular structure and higher fiber content. Not all complex carbohydrates are digested at the same rate.

Starchy Vegetables and other foods such as Refined Grains, Potatoes, Rice, and Grain-Based Flour generally cause a more rapid rise in blood sugar levels. This can be attributed to several factors, including their intrinsic molecular composition, the degree of processing and refinement they undergo, and how they are cooked and consumed.

Processing, Fiber, Fat/Protein, and Physical Form

Food Processing. Processed and refined carbohydrates are generally broken down more quickly than whole-food carbohydrates.

Presence of Fiber. Fiber can slow the digestion and absorption of carbohydrates, leading to a slower and steadier release of energy.

Fat and Protein. Consuming carbohydrates with fat and/or protein can slow their rate of digestion.

Physical Form. Liquid carbohydrates (like sugary drinks) tend to be absorbed more quickly than solid forms.

In Phase 2, we will connect how carbohydrates are digested with the effects that different carbohydrates have on your body so that you can take control and eat in harmony with how your body works. For now, keep in mind that some foods cause a fast rise in blood glucose, accompanied by a sharp rise in insulin, while other foods do not. Choosing foods that moderate the glucose and insulin response is at the heart of a sugar-free lifestyle. You will start by learning how to eliminate foods with added sugar in the following Action Steps.

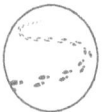

Action Steps

Read Labels to Find Added Sugar

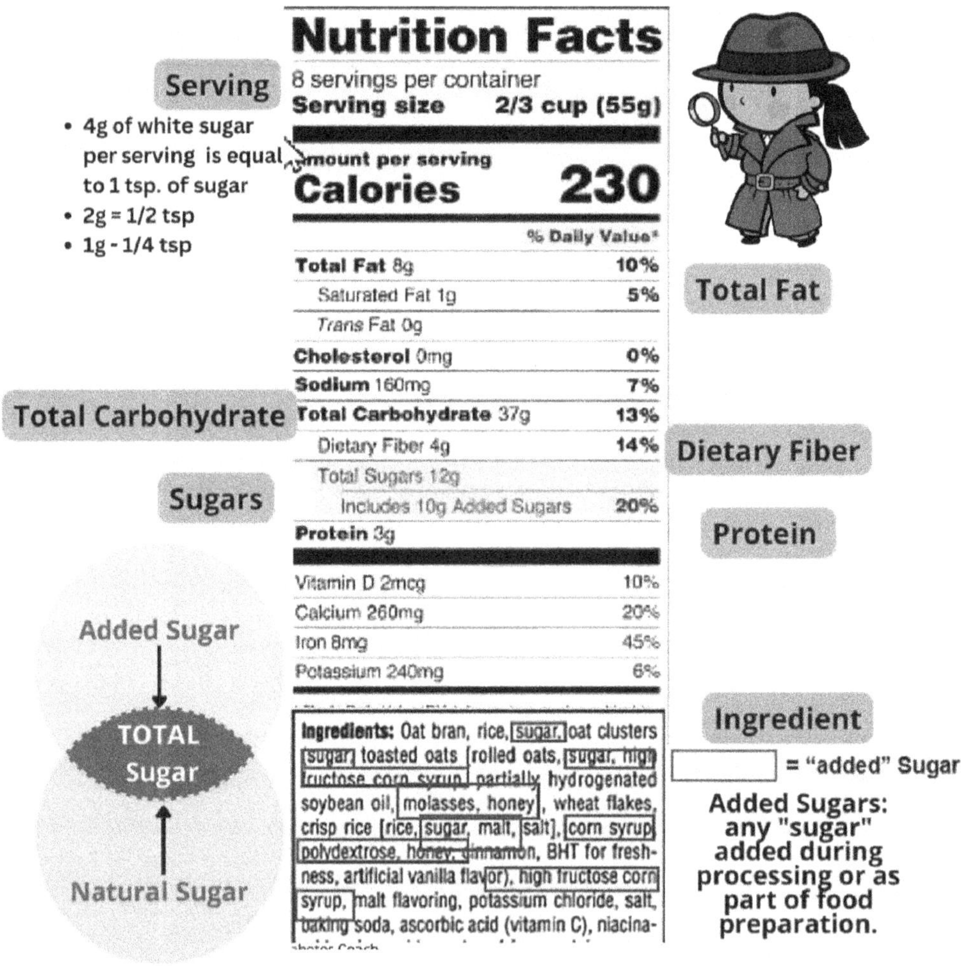

- Serving
  - 4g of white sugar per serving is equal to 1 tsp. of sugar
  - 2g = 1/2 tsp
  - 1g - 1/4 tsp

- Total Carbohydrate
- Sugars
- Added Sugar → TOTAL Sugar ← Natural Sugar
- Total Fat
- Dietary Fiber
- Protein
- Ingredient
  - ☐ = "added" Sugar
  - Added Sugars: any "sugar" added during processing or as part of food preparation.

- Food labels have a Nutrition Facts and an Ingredients section, which provide different types of information. Always read both the Nutrition Facts and Ingredients sections of the Food Label to understand the health value of a

food product. Together, they give you the TRUE picture of the food product's health and nutritional value.
- The FDA definition of "sugar," as found in the Code of Federal Regulations, means the natural sweet substance "obtained from sugar cane or sugar beets."
- The term "sugars" on a nutrition label means the sum of different types of sugars (such as glucose, fructose, lactose, and sucrose).
- The Nutrition Label contains a separate section for all sugars and for added sugars. The total sugar grams equal the sum of added sugars plus natural sugars.
- Added sugar is any sugar added during processing or as part of food preparation.
- Natural sugar means sugars that are found naturally in foods, such as lactose in dairy products, fructose in fruit, and maltose, which is found in a variety of foods, including grains.
- To find out if there is Added Sugar, you need to see if the label includes an Added Sugar amount. You also need to look at the ingredients section. A food that claims to have no added sugar means that NO sugar or ingredient containing sugar was added during processing or packaging, but it may still contain some natural sugar or artificial sweeteners.
- A food that claims it is Sugar-Free (a.k.a. zero sugar, sugarless) means that One Serving contains less than 0.5 grams of sugar (it might contain natural or added sugar).
- Ingredients are listed in order, starting with the ingredient found in the largest amount, by weight, and progressing to the ingredient present in the smallest amount.
- If you have type 2 diabetes and weigh about 140 pounds, 1 gram of pure glucose will raise your blood sugar by about 5 mg/dl—provided that your blood sugar is below the point at which your pancreas starts to make insulin to bring it down (1 Gram of granulated sugar is approximately equal to ¼ teaspoon (or ¼ sugar cube).
- Total Carbohydrate: This reflects the total amount of carbohydrates in the food product. In the nutrition facts table, the amount of total carbohydrates is the sum of sugar, starches, and dietary fiber. Although all sugars are classed as carbohydrates, not all carbohydrates are sugars.

The Many Names for Sugar on Food Labels

Sugar goes by many names. This makes it super easy for it to hide and often hard to find. What we know as "table sugar" or "sucrose" is actually a combination of two simple sugars: Glucose and Fructose.

- **Glucose** is transported to cells for use as energy via insulin. Some glucose is also stored in the liver as "glycogen" (a reserve that can be used by the body when glucose is low, such as during a fast). Insulin is also a fat storage hormone that stores excess glucose in the blood as fat.
- **Fructose** does not cause a direct rise in blood sugar levels because it goes directly to the liver, where it is processed into glucose, glycogen, or fatty acids.

More Names for Sugar		
Agave Nectar	Date Sugar	Maltose
Barbados sugar	Demerara sugar	Mannose
Barley malt	Dextrose	Maple syrup
Barley malt syrup	Fruit juice/Concentrate	Molasses
Beet sugar	Fructose	Muscovado
Brown sugar	Glucose	Palm sugar
Cane juice/Crystals	Golden sugar	Panocha
Cane sugar	Golden syrup	Powdered sugar
Caramel	Grape sugar	Raw sugar
Carob syrup	HFCS (high-fructose corn syrup)	Rice syrup
Castor sugar		Sorghum syrup
Coconut sugar	Honey	Sucrose
Confectioner's sugar	Malt syrup	Turbinado sugar
Corn syrup	Maltodextrin	
	Maltitol	

Avoid High Fructose Corn Syrup

There is one sweetener that many experts agree should be totally avoided, and that is high-fructose corn syrup (HFCS), which is an ingredient in many sweetened or processed foods. When corn is processed into HFCS, this sweetener is absorbed more quickly than regular sugar and enters your cells, becoming an uncontrolled source of carbon (acetyl-CoA) that is made into cholesterol and triglycerides. Additionally, none of the normal controls on appetite are triggered when you eat foods or beverages containing HFCS, so you tend to stay hungry and keep eating more sugar and refined foods, which continues to fuel this cycle.

Stop Adding Sugar to Food, Recipes, and Beverages

One of the most effective ways to reduce sugar intake is to stop adding sugar to foods and, in the process, recalibrating your taste buds.

Your taste buds are malleable and can adapt over time. When constantly exposed to high sugar levels, they become desensitized and need even more sugar to register the same level of sweetness. Conversely, when you decrease sugar intake, you'll initially find unsweetened foods less palatable, but your taste buds adjust over time. Soon, foods you once thought were not sweet enough will taste just right, and overly sweetened foods will seem excessively sugary.

Explore how food tastes without any added sugar, and use spices and natural flavoring extracts to add zip to your food. Coriander, nutmeg, ginger, cardamom, natural vanilla, and cinnamon are all spices that can make a dish taste sweeter and help satisfy your sweet tooth without adding any sugar. Almond, mint, maple, coconut, and lemon extracts can add flavor to everything from oatmeal to yogurt and sweet potato dishes.

Learn About Alternative Sweeteners

There is no easy or one-size-fits-all answer for how or when to use sugar substitutes. However, the natural desire for a sweet taste is something most of us have in common. And if ignored, for many people, it will end in cravings and binges.

Whether sugar substitutes work for you depends on your biochemistry and food triggers. Below is a summary of common natural sugar substitutes, as well as information about the sugar alcohol erythritol and artificial sweeteners such as aspartame and sucralose.

Stevia

Stevia is a non-caloric herbal extract derived from the leaves of the Stevia rebaudiana plant. The sweetness of stevia comes from compounds known as steviol glycosides. Stevia sweeteners contain one or more steviol glycosides. The types described below determine the taste and amount of sweetness.

- Stevioside is one of the most abundant glycosides in stevia leaves. Stevioside tends to have a slightly bitter aftertaste.
- Rebaudioside A (Reb A) is less bitter than Stevioside, making it a popular sweetener preparation option.
- Rebaudioside C, D, and E are less common and used to create products with improved taste and reduced bitterness.

Effect on Blood Sugars: In its pure form, Stevia has no calories and will not raise your blood glucose levels. Be aware, however, that some stevia products combine stevia leaf extract with other ingredients such as dextrose, maltodextrin, erythritol, or other fillers to help balance the sweetness of stevia and more closely mimic the taste or texture of sugar. If you're using a stevia-based substitute that's combined with other ingredients, you may still be getting some carbs and calories, and these products may raise your blood sugar levels.

Monk Fruit

Monk Fruit, also *known* as Luo Han Guo (or Siraitia grosvenorii), is a small, round fruit native to parts of Southeast Asia. Monk fruit naturally contains fructose and glucose, but when it's processed, the sugars are removed, and the remaining extract contains mogroside, which is the compound responsible for monk fruit's no-calorie sweetness. These compounds are extracted through a process that typically involves crushing the fruit and collecting the juice. The juice is then processed to isolate and purify the mogrosides, leaving behind a concentrated sweetener.

Effect on Blood Sugars: Like Stevia, in its pure form, Monk Fruit has no calories and will not raise your blood glucose levels. Also, like Stevia, some Monk Fruit products are combined with other ingredients such as dextrose, maltodextrin, or erythritol, and those products may raise your blood sugar levels. Some new products also combine Monk Fruit Extract with Allulose.

Allulose

Allulose is a rare sugar found naturally in certain foods, such as figs, raisins, and maple syrup. However, commercial production of allulose involves the enzymatic conversion of sugars like fructose from sources like corn or sugarcane. The process typically includes taking the fructose and then exposing it to an enzyme that converts the fructose structure into allulose. When consumed, allulose doesn't significantly raise blood glucose or insulin levels because humans lack the enzymes to fully break down allulose into energy. Instead, about 70-84% of ingested allulose is excreted unchanged in the urine. Allulose is sold on its own, and several companies are now creating alternative sweetener blends that contain allulose.

Agave Syrup

Agave Syrup is made through the extraction and purification of the juice of the agave cactus. It is mainly metabolized in the liver and has a lower glycemic index. It should, however, be used very sparingly because of its high fructose content. Consumption of high amounts of fructose triggers "lipogenesis," the process of converting excess carbohydrates into fatty acids in the liver and adipose tissue. These fatty acids can then be converted into triglycerides, such that excessive consumption of fructose can have a propensity to increase serum triglycerides. New studies are also showing a link between high fructose consumption and insulin resistance.

Sucralose

Sucralose, or SPLENDA® Brand Sweetener, is made from a patented multi-step process that begins with sugar (sucrose). Three hydrogen-oxygen groups on the sugar molecule are replaced with three chlorine atoms. Although the process of making sucralose begins with sugar, Sucralose is not recognized by the body as sugar or as a carbohydrate. It is not metabolized by the body for energy and does not affect blood glucose levels.

It should be noted that additional ingredients are added to SPLENDA® to give it volume and texture. These fillers include maltodextrin and/or dextrose, which contribute a small amount of calories per serving. (less than five calories). Although widely used in the United States, there is some controversy remaining over the safety of Splenda, which relates to the molecular makeup of sucralose. The sucralose molecule is an organochloride (or chlorocarbon). The root of the controversy is that while some industry experts claim the molecule is similar to table salt or sugar, other researchers claim that it has more in common with pesticides. That is because the bonds holding the carbon and chlorine atoms together are more characteristic of a chlorocarbon than a salt—and most pesticides are chlorocarbons.

Although some chlorocarbons are toxic, sucralose is not known to be toxic in small quantities and is extremely insoluble in fat; it cannot accumulate in fat like chlorinated hydrocarbons. In addition, sucralose does not break down or dechlorinate. So, the question remains: Is sucralose safe for everyday use? The answer is that we really don't know yet. The best advice is to use Splenda conservatively, in small amounts, if you would like to utilize it occasionally, and when possible, use other types of natural sugar substitutes.

Aspartame

Aspartame, the main ingredient in Equal and NutraSweet, may be responsible for the most serious adverse effects because the body digests it. Recent studies in Europe show that aspartame use can result in an accumulation of formaldehyde in the brain, which can damage your central nervous system and immune system and cause genetic trauma. The FDA admits this is true but claims the amount is low enough in most products that it shouldn't raise concern. The issue for consumers becomes: to what degree are we willing to risk our health by ingesting this potentially dangerous substance?

Aspartame has had the most complaints of any food additive available to the public. Possible side effects of aspartame include headaches, migraines, panic attacks, dizziness, irritability, nausea, intestinal discomfort, skin rash, and nervousness. Some researchers have linked aspartame with depression and manic episodes.

Sugar Alcohols: Mannitol, Maltitol, Sorbitol, and Xylitol

There are actually neither sugar nor alcohol, but they do have carbohydrate calories, approximately ½ to ¾ the calories of regular sugar. Derived from plant products, the carbohydrates are altered through a chemical process. They are more slowly and incompletely absorbed from the small intestine than sugar, thus producing a much smaller and slower rise in blood glucose levels and, consequently, also a smaller and slower rise in insulin. However, it should be noted that the rise in blood sugar differs depending on your individual makeup, and some of the sugar alcohols may have a laxative effect. When considering products with sugar alcohols, moderation is the key.

Erythritol

Erythritol is a "sugar alcohol" that is produced through a natural fermentation process. Erythritol also naturally occurs in minor amounts in fruits such as watermelon, pear, and grape, as well as fermented foods such as soy sauce and cheese. Most erythritol used as a sweetener in foods and beverages is produced synthetically. Erythritol has a minimal effect on blood sugar levels because, structurally, erythritol is a smaller molecule than other sugar alcohols. Even though a significant amount is absorbed into the blood (60 to 90%), it is then excreted in the urine. For this reason, erythritol generally does not cause the laxative effects often experienced after consumption of other sugar alcohols.

Up until recently, Erythritol was a popular sugar substitute for a variety of reasons. Recently, however, a study published in the journal Nature Medicine in February 2023 contains data that suggests a connection between erythritol and cardiovascular events such as clotting, stroke, and heart attacks.

The researchers recruited multiple groups of people with preexisting cardiac risk factors across the U.S. and Europe and tracked their health over time after taking blood samples to measure the amount of various compounds in the body. When looking at the data, the top-ranking compound found was erythritol. Of the 4,000 people included in the study's dataset, those who had high levels of erythritol in their blood were found to be more likely to suffer a major cardiac event within three years than those with lower levels. Additional lab and animal research presented in the paper revealed that erythritol appeared to be causing blood platelets to clot more readily.

All of this suggests using caution when it comes to using Erythritol as your sweetener of choice, although it is far from clear the degree to which Erythritol poses a health threat without further studies. Many sugar-free baking gurus routinely use(d) Erythritol in their recipes because of its qualities for good baking results. However, for other uses, such as sweetening beverages or sweetening non-baked desserts, sweeteners such as Stevia, Monk Fruit, and Allulose will work just as well.

Eliminate Soda, Including Diet

A growing body of research indicates that drinking artificially sweetened diet sodas on a regular basis may set you up for weight gain and cravings for sweets. New research suggests that the body learns to predict caloric intake by the taste and texture of certain foods. When artificial sweeteners are introduced into the mix, our body sends the appropriate sweet signals to the brain, but never delivers the sugar punch.

In this process, we set ourselves up for cravings to which we eventually and often unknowingly give in. In other words, consuming drinks that taste very sweet due to artificial sweeteners that seem real might be setting us up to eat more later on. An occasional diet soda is probably fine. But watch out for habitual drinking of artificially sweetened diet soda.

I recommend eliminating all regular and diet soda. But if you are currently drinking diet soda, don't feel like you have to go cold turkey, especially if that is going to set you up for failure. Create a plan for cutting back and work towards eliminating it from your food plan. Below are some steps you can take to cut back.

- Remove diet soda from your home environment. Don't keep it at your desk at work. Out of sight, out of mind.
- Set a rule for yourself that you will only drink diet soda when you're out at a restaurant or on an occasion outside of your home. Later, you can start substituting other drinks when you eat out until you're eventually soda-free.
- Be prepared for withdrawal symptoms. Your body is addicted to this substance. So don't be discouraged if you experience some physical effects of quitting that will subside, including headaches, irritability, or lack of focus.
- Time to quit so you can be out of focus and irritable without it affecting your life too much. Don't totally stop drinking diet soda the week you have major work deadlines or an important occasion on your calendar, such as a graduation, wedding, or other celebration. That's a recipe for disaster. Instead, cut back.

Water is the recommended liquid of choice. But if you are not a fan of plain water, there are many other options. As you review the suggestions below, remember to keep what you like and leave the rest. Everyone's biochemistry is different, and what may be fine for someone else might be a trigger food for you. Using a very small amount of sweeteners, such as Stevia or Monk Fruit, works for many people. For others, even a very small amount of sweet taste triggers cravings.

Tips and Ideas for Quitting Soda

- Flavor water or seltzer with Stevia or Monk Fruit drops, which are available in a variety of fruit and non-fruit flavors such as Vanilla or Root Beer.
- Unsweetened Tea is a good water alternative. If you enjoy iced tea, try making your own with decaf tea bags.
- Plain water is refreshing when infused with fruit such as strawberries, orange slices, lemons, limes, blueberries, or watermelon.
- A cup of hot chamomile tea at night is a relaxing way to end your day.
- You can also get water into your system from food sources, such as soups and vegetables that contain a high percentage of water.

Replace Salad Dressings that Contain Added Sugar

Once you have made an effort to create a delicious and satisfying salad, the last thing you want to do is pour a bunch of sugar over it and turn it into a blood sugar disaster. Store-bought dressings with no sugar added provide convenience, and you can use these dressings for all sorts of salads or as marinades. If you prefer homemade, below are some tips for making your own salad dressings and marinades.

Foolproof Dressing

Salad dressings generally have three major components: fat, acid, and an emulsifier (which combines the two). Mustard, mayonnaise, tahini, and mashed avocado are common emulsifiers for homemade salad dressings.

- A foolproof way to "dress" your salad is to drizzle a small amount of extra-virgin olive oil over the greens and mix it in well. The greens should be lightly dressed, not soggy.
- Then, add a small amount of your choice of vinegar or lemon juice to taste. Finally, add some seasonings. My favorite combo is lemon-flavored olive oil with fruit-flavored balsamic vinegar.
- When the salad dressing is applied and mixed using this method, you don't need to add an emulsifier unless you want to do so for extra flavor.

Quick Tricks for Extra Flavor

- Whether making your own or using a bottled dressing, you don't want a soggy salad. Start with a small amount, mix and coat the salad, and then add more to taste, if needed.
- To add amazing flavor to an otherwise "bland dressing," add a variety of very finely chopped vegetables (carrots, peppers, onions, celery, whatever you have on hand). I love to add finely chopped veggies to Newman's Own Oil and Vinegar dressing to give it a little "kick." The only time-consuming part is chopping the vegetables, although you can find them already chopped as "mirepoix" in most grocery stores.

Replace Yogurt Containing Added Sugar with Plain Yogurt (and Flavor the Yogurt Yourself)

Yogurt is often touted as a healthy snack packed with probiotics, protein, and essential nutrients like calcium and vitamin D. However, not all yogurts are created equal, and the difference often lies in the plain versus flavored products. One of the most significant advantages of choosing plain yogurt is its lower sugar content. Flavored yogurts often contain added sugars that can quickly turn your healthy snack into a sugar-laden choice.

Plain yogurt, on the other hand, contains natural sugars found in milk and has no added sugars. The more lactose in the yogurt, the greater the amount of natural sugars. Plain yogurt acts as a blank canvas, allowing you to personalize your yogurt experience to your liking.

Ideas to "Jazz" Up Plain Yogurt

- Sweeten with flavored Stevia or Monk Fruit Drops
- Swirl in berries or make a berry parfait
- Add flavors such as Vanilla and/or Cinnamon
- Make a pudding with Cacao Powder and Protein Powder
- Thicken and add creaminess with Whipped Cream, Ricotta, or Mascarpone
- Top with Chopped Nuts, Chia Seeds, or Sugar-Free Chocolate Chips

Replace High Sugar Smoothies with No Added Sugar/Low Natural Sugar Alternatives

The trick to making smoothies for blood sugar health is combining a blend of low-sugar ingredients that will provide lots of nutrients and not cause major blood sugar and insulin spikes. The key ingredients for a delicious and healthy smoothie are:

Liquid + Protein + Fiber + Low Glycemic Fruits and/or Vegetables + Thickener + Sweetener of Choice.

Smoothie Formula

THICKENER
- Ice
- Frozen Berries
- Frozen Cauliflower
- 1/4 Frozen Banana (less ripe)
- Avocado, Tofu, Yogurt, Mascarpone, Chia Seeds will also serve as thickeners

OTHER
- Greens Powder
- Acai Powder
- Goji Berry Powder
- Cinnamon
- Vanilla Flavoring
- Cacao Nibs
- Cacao Powder

LIQUID
- Dairy Milk
- Nut Milk (Unsweetened)
- Coconut Milk (Unsweetened)
- Soy Milk
- Kefir
- Water
- Coffee

FRUIT/VEGETABLES
- Acai (Unsweetened)
- Berries (Strawberries, Blueberry, Raspberry, Blackberry)
- 1/4 Banana (less ripe)
- Frozen Cauliflower
- Kale/Spinach
- Pumpkin/Squash
- Carrots

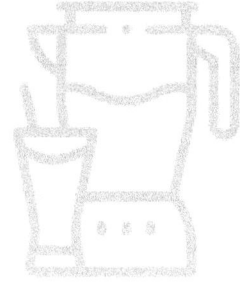

PROTEIN/FIBER
- Protein Powder
- Silken Tofu
- Plain Yogurt
- Mascarpone
- Ground Flax Seeds
- Chia Seeds
- Almond Butter
- Peanut Butter

SWEETENERS
- Stevia Powder or Flavored Stevia Drops
- Monk Fruit Powder or Flavored Drops
- Choc Zero Syrups
- Wholesome Yum Zero Sugar Honey
- Other Non-Sugar Sweetener of Choice

Replace Pantry Items (Such as Condiments, Canned Goods, and Processed Foods) with Brands Containing No Added Sugar

Examples of foods that are easy to replace with a no-sugar-added brand include:

- Pasta Sauce
- Vinegar
- Peanut Butter/Almond Butter
- Protein Powder
- Maple Syrup & Honey
- Salad Dressings
- Mayonnaise

- Chocolate (Dark Chocolate & Cacao Powder)
- Prepared Soup
- Pancake Mixes
- Ice Cream
- Yogurt
- Dairy Alternatives (Examples: Almond, Oat, Coconut, Milks)

No Added Sugar Substitution Ideas

The following suggestions are for products that were available at the time this book was published. Everyone's tastes are different, and some may be right for you, while others may not. The purpose of the list is to give you ideas and help you get started.

Salad Dressings and Marinades

Homemade or bottled No Sugar Added alternatives such as:

- Newman's Own: Classic Oil & Vinegar Dressing, Creamy Caesar Dressing
- Annie's: Organic Goddess Dressing, Organic Red Wine & Olive Oil Vinaigrette
- Tessemae's: Organic Lemon Garlic Dressing, Classic Italian
- Primal Kitchen: Ranch, Lemon Turmeric Vinaigrette
- Drew's: Organic Shitake Ginger Dressing, Tahini Goddess Dressing, Classic Italian
- Sir Kensington Dressings
- Cindy's Kitchen Barcelona Vinaigrette
- Trader Joe's Organic Red Wine & Olive Oil Vinaigrette

Ketchup, Mayonnaise, and Salsa

- Ketchup: Heinz No Sugar Added Ketchup, Primal Kitchen Unsweetened Ketchup
- Mayonnaise: Dukes Real Mayonnaise, 365 by Whole Foods Market
- Salsa: Newman's Own, Pace, Tostitos, Siete, Nature's Promise (Organic)

Chocolate & Cacao/Cocoa Powder

- Chocolate: Lily's, ChocZero, Lakanto (small amounts, watch portion sizes of chocolate with Erythritol)
- Cacao Powder: Navitas (Organic) Better Body Foods (Organic)
- Cocoa Powder: Ghirardelli, Now Real Food (Organic)

Pancakes

- Birch Benders Keto Pancake & Waffle Mix

Waffles

- Chaffles (made with eggs and cream cheese or various types of cheeses)

Maple Syrup

- Birch Benders Keto Syrup
- ChocZero No Sugar Maple Syrup
- Wholesome Yum Zero Sugar Maple Syrup
- Lakanto Maple Flavored Syrup

Honey

- Wholesome Yum Zero Sugar Honey Substitute

Whey Powder

- Ascent 100% Whey (Native Whey Protein Blend), 365 Whey Isolate Protein (Unflavored), Levels Whey Protein Powder

Ice Cream

- Yogurt or Ricotta "pudding"
- No Added Sugar Ice Cream Brands (no sorbitol or maltitol): Halo Top, So Delicious, Rebel, Nicks, Keto Pint

Plain Yogurt

- Greek: Fage (Plain and Lactose Free Plain), Stonyfield Organic, Chobani, Maple Hill Creamery
- Icelandic Skyr: Siggi's, Icelandic Provisions

- Coconut: So Delicious, Cocojune, Coconut Cult,
- Almond: Kite Hill Unsweetened, DAH!, Silk Unsweetened

Cereal and Granola

- Catalina Crunch Keto Cereal, Magic Spoon Keto Cereal
- Magic Spoon No-Grain Granola

Peanut Butter, Almond Butter

- Peanut Butter: Justins, MaraNatha
- Almond Butter: Kirkland No Added Sugar, Good & Gather Unsweetened Almond Butter, 365 Organic Almond Butter, Maranatha No Added Sugar or Salt No Stir Almond Butter

Pasta Sauce:

- Rao's Homemade, Classico, Target Good & Gather, Primal Kitchen

Takeaways & Highlights

The phase of change called Adapting is the bridge between the old and the new, where you give yourself the time and space to start taking action, learn from your experiences, and build resilience.

A foundation for living a sugar-free lifestyle is eliminating added sugar. You can begin to find and replace added sugar with the following Action Steps.

- Read Labels to Find Added Sugar
- Stop Adding Sugar to Food, Recipes, and Beverages
- Learn About Alternative Sweeteners
- Eliminate Soda (including diet)
- Replace Salad Dressings that Contain Added Sugar
- Replace Yogurt Containing Added Sugar with Plain Yogurt (and Flavor the Yogurt Yourself)

- Replace High Sugar Smoothies with No Added Sugar/Low Natural Sugar Alternatives
- Replace Pantry Items (such as condiments, canned goods, and prepared foods) with brands containing no Added Sugar.

Following a particular order when engaging in the find and replace added sugar activities is not required. I recommend starting with "Find Added Sugar" and "Stop Adding Sugar to Food, Recipes, and Beverages."

Carbohydrates are not a food. They are a collection of carbon, oxygen, and hydrogen molecules.

- A single carbohydrate molecule is called a "saccharide," a fancy word for a sugar molecule.
- Carbohydrates are classified into several different types based on the number of sugar molecules they contain, and each type metabolizes in our body differently.
- The four types of carbohydrates include Monosaccharides (single sugar unit), Disaccharides (two sugar units), Oligosaccharides (3-10 sugar units), and Polysaccharides (more than ten simple sugar units and sometimes up to thousands).
- Polysaccharides are ultimately broken down into Monosaccharide sugar units (Glucose, Fructose, Galactose) during the digestion process.

Not all carbohydrates are processed in the same way. Some foods cause a fast rise in blood glucose accompanied by a sharp rise in insulin, while other foods do not.

- The amount of carbohydrates consumed and the rate at which the processed sugar enters our bloodstream affect blood sugar levels, cravings, and how fat is stored in our bodies.
- Rapid absorption can lead to swift spikes in blood sugar levels accompanied by a sharp rise in insulin, especially if consumed in large quantities or without other macronutrients like fiber, protein, or fat.

Learning how to choose foods that moderate the glucose and insulin response is at the heart of living a sugar-free lifestyle.

CHAPTER 10
Gain Clarity (Where You Are and Where You Want to Go) to Embark on a New Beginning

Coach on Your Shoulder

In prior chapters, we explored how commitment, connection, and consistent action help you to adapt to new foods and behaviors. In this chapter, you will learn about the connection between gaining clarity and embarking on a new beginning to create a lasting sugar-free lifestyle.

Clarity and New Beginnings

A fine line exists between endings, beginnings, and the period of adapting.

Genuine new beginnings are heralded by a shift in attitude. Along with a renewal of energy, there is a deeper sense of knowing where you want to go, even if you don't yet have a total plan in place for how you will get there. Developing clarity about where you are and where you want to go provides the springboard that empowers you to create your action plan and launches you toward new ways of eating and creating a sugar-free lifestyle.

Embarking on a new beginning does not mean that you will never have setbacks or that you have all the answers. The hallmark of embarking on a new beginning is that you have a clearer connection to self, and you are no longer motivated by a set of external "shoulds" thrust upon you by doctors, experts, or well-meaning friends or relatives. Instead, your motivation comes from within, driven by your goals, individual needs, and vision for your future.

Clarity is not something that happens overnight. It is an ongoing process that is built into each step of the Sugar-Free Lifestyle Roadmap™. The purpose of this chapter is to help you understand the importance of self-awareness and to explain the various activities and worksheets that are provided throughout this book.

It is not necessary to complete all the worksheets and activities in this chapter before moving on to Phases 2 and 3. However, you can return to this Chapter anytime you feel stuck or want to revisit your current state of physical, mental, or spiritual well-being, so that you can keep your day-to-day decisions aligned with your goals and vision of health.

Key Concepts

Levels of Clarity: Where Am I and Where Do I Want to Go?

Below is a diagram illustrating the levels of clarity and the tools you can use throughout your journey to clarify your vision, set goals, and develop your action plan.

The first step in changing behavior is self-awareness, which is having a conscious knowledge of yourself at several levels: physically, mentally, and spiritually. Gaining self-awareness requires the ability to monitor and pay attention to your present environment and experience. This is often called being "in the moment."

There are two aspects of self-awareness: knowing where you are now and where you want to go in the future. Clarity about your present state serves as the foundation for your vision of the future.

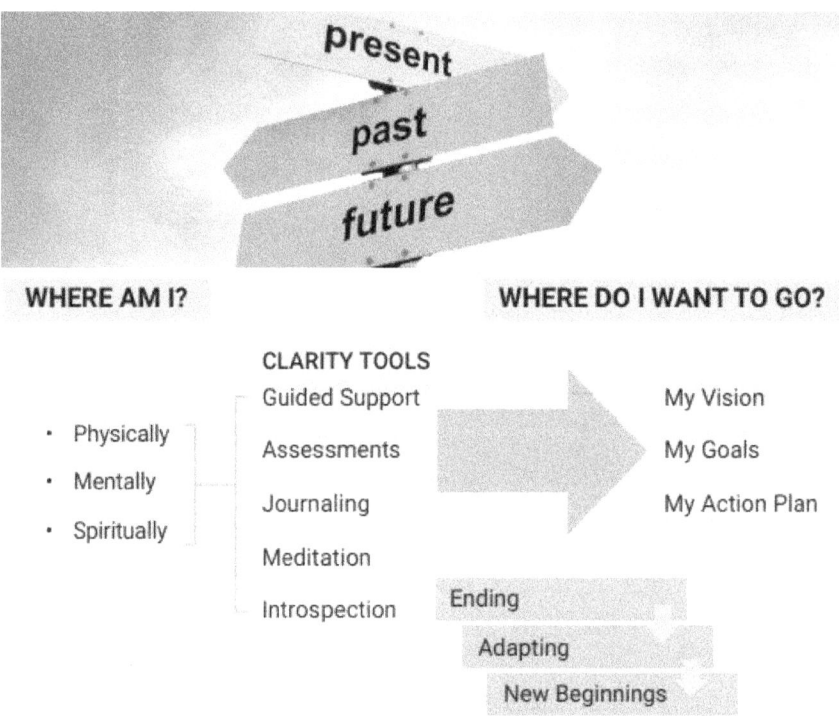

Many people rush into their action steps without taking the time to develop the clarity that is needed for future success. Moving forward without clarity is like fumbling around in a dark room filled with obstacles, getting nowhere, and feeling lots of pain. The benefits of having clarity relating to your present circumstances and your vision for the future include:

- Enabling you to identify and address roadblocks, thoughts, and behaviors holding you back.
- Giving you deeper insight so that you can make decisions that are right for you based on your unique vision of health, life goals, and bio-individuality.
- Shedding light on your "why" so that when the going gets tough, you will have the internal motivation that will enable you to keep moving forward.
- Providing critical insights that shape your goals and action plan.

Health Tests to Find Out Where You Are Physically

Before you start any program, it is a good idea to get a handle on where you are physically for a variety of reasons. Most importantly, you want to make sure that any decisions you make will not exacerbate any underlying conditions that you may not be aware of and that you are aligning your action plan with your physical state and unique biochemistry.

If you are worried about insulin resistance, pre-diabetes, or diabetes, below are four tests to discuss with your physician that will help you determine whether you have any of these conditions. This is important because your physical state has a direct impact on your food choices.

- **Fasting Plasma Glucose.** After an 8 to 12-hour fast, your blood is drawn and blood sugar levels measured. Per new ADA guidelines, a reading of less than 100 mg/dl is normal; 100 to 125 indicates pre-diabetes, and 126 or higher is a sign of full-blown diabetes.
- **Oral Glucose Tolerance Test**. During this test, your blood sugar is measured after a fast and then again 2 hours after drinking a beverage containing a large amount of glucose. Two hours after the drink, if your glucose is higher than normal, you have what's called "impaired glucose tolerance" ("IGT").
- HbA1c Screening Test: This is a blood test that measures the level of Hemoglobin A1C in your blood. It is utilized to indicate your average blood glucose over a 2-3 month period. According to ADA recommendations, a normal HbA1c level is less than 6% for nondiabetics, and a GOAL for diabetics is less than 7%. Studies show that people with diabetes who keep their A1C levels below 7% are less likely to develop diabetic complications.
- **Thyroid Testing**. The thyroid is the body's accelerator, controlling the tempo of all its internal processes. When the gland doesn't work hard enough, a condition called hypothyroidism develops. When it starts to work too hard, hyperthyroidism develops.
    - o A TSH test can be taken to determine if your thyroid is working properly. This test measures thyroid-stimulating hormone made by the pituitary gland to keep the thyroid under control. Criteria vary,

but a TSH higher than 5 mIU/ml usually indicates hypothyroidism, and a TSH below 0.1 indicates hyperthyroidism.
- o I included thyroid testing in this section because both hypothyroidism and hyperthyroidism significantly impact metabolism and energy levels. Hypothyroidism, characterized by an underactive thyroid gland, leads to a slower metabolism, often causing fatigue, weight gain, and decreased appetite. Conversely, hyperthyroidism involves an overactive thyroid, which accelerates metabolism, which can result in increased energy, weight loss, heightened appetite, and cravings. Both conditions disrupt normal metabolic processes, affecting overall energy balance and contributing to changes in body weight, hunger, and food cravings.
- o Thyroid disease can be challenging to diagnose by symptoms alone because many other illnesses cause the same symptoms. If you have glucose imbalances or diabetes, you are at higher risk for thyroid disease. If you are experiencing any of the symptoms described above, talk to your doctor about testing. After testing, if your TSH test is within normal ranges, but your symptoms persist, you should consider speaking to your physician about testing the levels of the T4 and T3 thyroid hormones in your blood.

Tests Your Heart Will Love You For

Insulin resistance, pre-diabetes, and diabetes are closely interconnected conditions that significantly increase the risk of heart disease. Insulin resistance occurs when cells become less responsive to insulin, leading to elevated blood sugar levels. This can progress to pre-diabetes, where blood sugar levels are higher than normal but not yet high enough to be classified as diabetes. If untreated, pre-diabetes often leads to type 2 diabetes, characterized by consistently high blood sugar levels.

All these conditions can contribute to the development of cardiovascular complications, including heart disease, due to the damaging effects of high blood sugar on blood vessels and the increased risk of atherosclerosis. Regular checkups and testing are crucial for early detection and management, helping to prevent the progression of insulin resistance to diabetes and reduce the risk of heart disease through timely intervention and lifestyle modifications.

Below are some tests to be aware of. I have provided general guidelines for recommended test levels. However, these guidelines do not replace medical care. You should confirm the meaning of your test results with your physician, who can provide information in the context of your specific results and follow up with next steps.

- **Total Cholesterol**. Cholesterol is a waxy substance produced by the liver or supplied in the diet, through animal products such as meat, poultry, fish and dairy products. Cholesterol does not dissolve in the blood, so it must be carried through the bloodstream by proteins, called lipoproteins. It is generally recommended that total cholesterol be less than 200 mg/dL.
- **Low-Density Lipoprotein (LDL)**. LDL carries cholesterol through the blood and is often called the "bad" cholesterol. When there is too much LDL cholesterol in the blood, it combines with other substances to form deposits on the blood vessel walls. This causes a narrowing of the blood vessels and increases the risk of heart attack. It is generally recommended that LDL be less than 100 mg/dL.
- **High-Density Lipoprotein (HDL)**. Often called the "good" cholesterol, HDL removes cholesterol from the blood vessel walls and carries it back to the liver to be disposed of. HDL cholesterol can be raised by regular exercise or weight loss. It can also be improved by consuming a daily diet low in sugar, starch, and trans-fat. It is generally recommended that HDL be greater than 4o mg/dL (Men) or greater than 55 mg/dL (Women).
- **LDL-P**. Cholesterol is a fatty oil that can't travel around in your bloodstream on its own. It needs to be packed into what are known as "particles." The particles are what deliver the bad cholesterol inside the walls of the artery to form plaque, and the more particles you have, the greater your risk for heart disease. This number is known as LDL-P, and you want this number to be less than 1000. Small dense particles are more likely to damage our artery wall as they can enter more easily than larger LDL particles. So, you also want to

include testing for levels of sd-LDL to understand if you have a large number of small dense LDL particles.
- **LP(a):**. Another type of cholesterol you might want to be aware of, especially if you have diabetes or pre-diabetes, is Lp(a) cholesterol. With an attached "corkscrew" called apoprotein (a), Lp(a) is an inherited trait that can increase risk of heart disease and stroke. Having high levels of this form of LDL can be unnerving because there is very little that can be done in terms of lifestyle to bring Lp(a) down. But the good news is that being even more vigilant with your other lipid numbers can help with your overall risk for heart disease. If you are diabetic or pre-diabetic, it is important to work with your doctor to make sure you are getting the tests you need to understand where you are and what you need to do to manage your heart health.
- **Triglycerides** are a combination of three fatty acids found in the foods we eat. Insulin allows triglycerides to enter the fat cells for storage. If this process does not take place properly and the triglycerides stay in the bloodstream, this can lead to heart disease. It is generally recommended that triglyceride levels be less than 150.
- **Homocysteine Levels**. Homocysteine is an amino acid produced by the metabolic breakdown of methionine, an essential component of dietary protein. Recent studies indicate that elevated levels of homocysteine may be an independent risk factor for cardiovascular disease.
- **C-Reactive Protein**: Another factor that may point to heart disease is a higher level of C-reactive protein, which is produced by the liver and fat cells. Its level dramatically increases when there is inflammation anywhere in the body. The higher the CRP, the greater the chance of a plaque rupturing and causing a heart attack. One thing to remember is that CRP can be elevated for several reasons. If you are at risk for heart disease, consult your physician about having your CRP levels tested.
- **Fibrinogen**. This is a sticky, fibrous protein substance manufactured by your liver that promotes clotting and is part of the body's natural repair system. A certain level of fibrinogen is essential, and at normal levels, fibrinogen performs necessary and important functions in the human body. However, too high levels can make the blood thicker and make it more difficult for the heart to pump this

thicker blood through the whole body. There is also greater chance of forming a clot that can obstruct an artery. Many studies have shown that elevated fibrinogen is a risk factor for heart attacks and strokes. The normal range for fibrinogen is 200 - 400 milligrams per deciliter (mg/dL).

- **Blood Pressure Monitoring**. Blood pressure is the measure of the force exerted by the circulating blood on the walls of your arteries. It is expressed by two numbers: systolic pressure (the top number, which measures the pressure exerted on the arteries during a contraction of the heart when the heart pumps blood out of the chambers) and diastolic pressure (the bottom number, which measures the amount of pressure exerted when your heart relaxes and the chambers fill-up with blood). High blood pressure occurs when the force required to pump blood through the arteries increases due to a narrowing of the blood vessels. The latest ADA guidelines for diabetics recommend that BP should be controlled to less than 140/90 mm/Hg or 130/80 mm/Hg if a higher risk of cardiovascular disease exists.
- **Intima Media Thickness Scanning (IMT)**. This is a non-invasive scanning technique used to measure the thickness of the inner layer of the carotid artery wall. This test is used to determine the extent of plaque buildup in the walls of the arteries that supply blood to the head and is an independent predictor of TIA (stroke-like symptoms), stroke, and heart disease.

Tests to Keep Your Body Parts Intact

Diabetes complications such as retinopathy, neuropathy, and kidney disease arise from prolonged high blood sugar levels, which damage blood vessels and nerves throughout the body. Diabetic retinopathy affects the eyes, potentially leading to vision loss, while neuropathy causes nerve damage, resulting in pain, tingling, and loss of sensation, particularly in the extremities. Kidney disease, or nephropathy, impairs kidney function, which can lead to kidney failure.

Maintaining a sugar-free lifestyle is an integral part of avoiding diabetes complications. However, regular testing is still crucial to detect these complications early, allowing for timely treatment and management. Early detection through regular eye exams, nerve function tests, and kidney function tests can help prevent or slow the progression of these severe complications, improving quality of life and reducing the risk of long term damage. Below are three tests that should be discussed with your medical team.

- **Dilated Retinal Eye Exam**. Over time, diabetes can damage the tiny blood vessels of the retina (a light-sensitive tissue in the back of the eye that receives and transmits focused images to the brain), and abnormal blood vessel growth may occur. This condition is called Diabetic Retinopathy, a complication of diabetes. Retinopathy can be detected through a dilated eye exam performed by an optometrist or an ophthalmologist.
- **Foot Exams**. Peripheral neuropathy (nerve damage in the legs and feet) and vascular disease (poor circulation) are major factors contributing to diabetic foot problems. Together, these problems make it easy to get ulcers and infections that, without care, could lead to amputations. The best defense against these complications is tight glucose control, taking good care of your feet, and seeing your physician right away if foot problems arise.
- **Microalbumin Measurement**. This is a test that measures small amounts of protein in your urine. This test is important because diabetes can damage the tiny blood-filtering units in your kidneys, where waste products from your blood are removed and eliminated in your urine. This allows protein molecules in your blood, such as albumin, to leak into the urine. There are no early symptoms, but your doctor can determine the presence and extent of early kidney disease by measuring the amount of protein in your urine.

Gaining Clarity About Primary and Secondary Foods

We nourish our bodies in many different ways. An important aspect of self-awareness relates not only to understanding your physical state and nutritional habits, but also to gaining clarity about your mental, emotional, and spiritual well-being. This includes understanding where you are in terms of your career, physical activity, and relationships.

When I was a student at The Institute for Integrative Nutrition, Joshua Rosenthal, founder of IIN, referred to these as "primary foods." Primary foods are your dreams and the things that feed your spirituality, whereas secondary foods are what you eat to nourish your body. Many people choose to eat certain secondary foods in an attempt to influence how they are feeling, and the food we eat is intricately related to our mental, emotional, and spiritual state. Emotional and stress eating can be powerful forces that hinder cutting sugar, maintaining a blood sugar-friendly food plan, and achieving other life goals.

That is why it is essential to have clarity about your current state in terms of both primary and secondary foods in order to make a comprehensive action plan for vibrant health. Practically speaking, this means identifying how you feel about what you eat, when you eat, and patterns that indicate whether you are using food as a way to calm your emotions or cope with stress. In this chapter's Action Steps and the remaining chapters, we will explore how you can identify the triggers that lead to emotional and stress eating and how to break free from eating patterns that sabotage your efforts.

Why Your Action Plan is a Major Key to Success

Through counseling clients over the years, I have learned that most of us can learn what to do to maintain a sugar-free lifestyle. The difficulty arises when trying to implement necessary changes and adhering to them into the future. Without consistent action, knowledge will not take you very far. When you are ready to embark on a new beginning, creating an action plan is an essential step.

The foundation for an effective action plan is having clarity about your current state, a vision for the future, and the goals you want to achieve. Your action plan provides you with the specific activities and habits you will implement to achieve your sugar-free lifestyle and health goals.

When you are having difficulties, your action plan is a tool that you can rely on to reinforce positive lifestyle choices. Life is messy. The best intentions can go awry. If you don't exercise for a couple of days or some French fries get the best of you, don't panic or berate yourself. When you find yourself going off-track you can use your written action plan to GET BACK TO BASICS.

Creating Action Plans Based on Your Goals and Vision

Action plans move you forward by providing clear goals and specific activities to help you achieve your objectives. As you gain clarity about both your primary and secondary foods, you may discover that you have goals related explicitly to quitting sugar and others that are tangential to living a sugar-free lifestyle. These life goals are very often the foundation of your "why" for going sugar-free.

Here are some examples of short-term and long-term goals:

- Quitting all added sugar in 3 months
- Lose 20 pounds and gain more lean muscle mass in 6 months
- Go back to school within the next 6 months and complete a degree in psychology in 4 years.
- Take a cooking class within the next year and learn how to cook and plan vegetarian, sugar-free meals.
- Move to California within 5 years and live in a town with a vibrant, health-conscious community.
- Update my kitchen within 1 year to include a new stove and pantry to organize my food and kitchen staples.

Don't get overly concerned if you're not ready to create a comprehensive action plan. I have structured the chapters and activities throughout this book to guide you through this process, and you can always revisit activities that you are not yet ready to tackle. Follow along, and all will be revealed.

To this end, the Action Steps in this chapter provide guidance and worksheets for creating your vision, setting goals, and identifying activities to develop an action plan for achieving your objectives.

Creating your vision and setting goals is a process. You do not need to know all of your goals to progress to Phases 2 and 3, and both your vision and goals will likely evolve as you move forward. You can return to your Action Step worksheets at any time and update them as your self-knowledge and life circumstances change.

The Roadmap Action Plan

PHASE ONE: Embrace Change to Break Free From Sugar

- Commit to Making Lasting Changes and Adopting the 4 C's of Change and Resilience
- Connect to Yourself and a Supportive Community to Let Go of the Past
- Consistently Take Action to Quit Sugar and Adapt to a Sugar-Free Lifestyle
- Gain Clarity (Where You Are and Where You Want to Go) to Embark on a New Beginning

PHASE TWO: Nourish Your Body to LIVE Free from Sugar

- Learn How Your Body Works: The Sugar, Mind, and Body Connection
- Implement a Food Plan that Eliminates Personal Trigger Foods
- Validate, Monitor, and Adjust Your Plan
- Enhance Your Food Plan with Exercise, Restful Sleep, and Stress Management

PHASE THREE: Transform Your Mind To STAY FREE from Sugar

- Find the Thoughts, Roadblocks, and Eating Patterns Getting in Your Way
- Reverse Sabotaging Thoughts, Habits, and Eating Patterns
- Eliminate Clutter in Your Space to Create an Environment that Supports Lasting Change
- Enjoy Life!

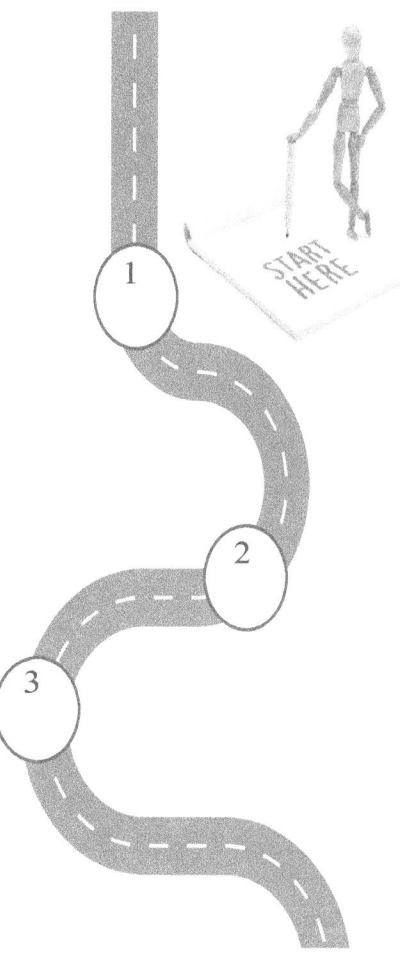

How to Develop Your Vision

In order to develop an effective plan for conquering sugar or managing any chronic health condition, it is essential to first have a clear vision of your future that will propel you towards your goals. Your unique vision serves as the foundation for your action plan and provides the motivation needed to keep moving forward when life gets in the way.

Your vision is not just about what you will eat. It will also include other hopes and aspirations relating to your life's work, recreation, physical activity, and relationships. These are your dreams that feed your spirit and help you to stay motivated.

One way to think about your life vision is to identify qualities you would like to develop, things you would like to do, and things you would like to have as a healthy person living a sugar-free lifestyle. Part of your vision will be directly related to your food plan and physical health, while other aspects will include things you hope to achieve as part of your overall life plan. Below are some examples:

QUALITIES I WOULD LIKE TO DEVELOP:

- I would like to be more energetic
- I would like to be more focused
- I would like to be physically fit

THINGS I WOULD LIKE TO DO:

- I would like to go back to school and learn how to be a chef
- I would like to take a year off from work and travel
- I would like to write a book

THINGS I WOULD LIKE TO HAVE:

- I would like to have a home in the country with a family and two dogs
- I would like to have a vegetable garden
- I would like to have more friends and time to spend with them

The Importance of Setting Goals as the Foundation for Your Action Plan

Setting goals and then accomplishing them with an action plan is crucial for improving your health and accomplishing what you want in your personal life. There is a direct relationship between goals and achievements because:

- Well-defined goals provide direction and help you achieve your desired results,
- Written goals provide you with a means of measuring progress,
- Setting priorities keeps you focused and moving ahead on a steady path, and
- Your progress in working towards your goals provides you with a source of information that can be used to adjust ongoing behaviors so that you can fine-tune your efforts and attain success.

The goal-setting process should ultimately:

- Identify long and short-term goals, which are broken down into manageable sub-parts so that progress can be measured,
- Provide a framework that will assist you in identifying priorities and activities to help you reach your goals,
- Set forth reasonably attainable goals as well as goals that are a stretch so that you will experience ongoing positive feedback and a sense of accomplishment and
- Provide you with a source of information that can be used to monitor and adjust ongoing behaviors.

Reviewing goals regularly makes it easier for you to fine-tune your efforts and helps you identify non-productive activities that can be abandoned. It is not necessary to be perfect as you work through your action plan.

Think of your goals as miles traveled on a winding road that will lead you to your destination. At times, you may find yourself on the side of the road. But, as long as you keep the road you have chosen in sight, you can get back to it at your own pace, and you will ultimately reach the goals you have set for yourself. The information on the following pages will describe what is involved in the goal-setting process and how to develop a set of goals that support your life vision.

THE ANATOMY OF A GOAL

✓ The goal is written, measurable and has a deadline

GOAL: Lose 30 lbs in 5 months

✓ The goal is broken down into reasonable sub-goals

SUB - GOAL: Lose 10 lbs in 1st 30 days (1 month)

SUB - GOAL: Lose 10 lbs in next 60 days (2 months)

SUB - GOAL: Lose 10 lbs in next 60 days (2 months)

✓ Activities are identified to lead you towards your goal (along with identifying obstacles to completing those activities & completion strategies)

Develop Food Plan & Follow Daily

Change My Plate (50% Non-starchy veggies, 25% Protein, 25% Healthy Fats & Other)

Exercise 30 minutes (aerobic) 6 days per week

How to Turn Written Goals Into Action

- **Identify your goals and put them in writing**. Articulating long-term and short-term goals and putting them in writing provides clarity and demonstrates a commitment to achieving your goals. Goals that stay in your head usually become confusing and are easily abandoned. Written goals tend to be more specific than unwritten goals and are more likely to be achieved.
- **Divide your goals into sub-goals**. These are steps or achievements you will strive to accomplish on the way to achieving the main goal. Subgoals provide an objective method of measuring your progress toward the main goal and show you where you may have to make adjustments. Achieving

sub-goals also provides you with a sense of confidence that will encourage you to keep moving forward toward the attainment of your ultimate goal.

- **Define activities to help you take consistent actions toward your goals.** Defining specific activities enables you to take action and move consistently toward your goals. These activities become the building blocks that are the foundation for your goals and the criteria for measuring your progress.

- **Identify any obstacles that you perceive as getting in your way of achieving your goals and, ultimately, your life vision.** Ask yourself if any obstacles stand in your way of achieving your goals, and identify solutions that will help you move forward. If you have beliefs that are holding you back, now is the time to uncover the roots of those beliefs so that you can move past them.

- **Establish reasonable deadlines for achieving your goals.** Setting deadlines provides closure and ensures that a particular goal does not remain unattended for too long a time period. Too many open-ended activities can be frustrating, leaving one with a sense of not getting anything done.

- **Learn to distinguish goals from open-ended desires.** If you have trouble committing a goal to writing, it probably isn't a goal but an open-ended desire (that you may or may not be able to translate into a goal). Sometimes, as you attempt to list the activities that will help you achieve a particular goal, you may find that you simply do not want to engage in those activities. When this happens, you may decide to postpone that goal or abandon it altogether.

- **Take daily consistent action to achieve your goals.** The activities that you defined are the fuel to propel you toward creating and maintaining a sugar-free lifestyle. If you fall, you can get up. If you find yourself going off track, you can use your activities as a compass to guide you toward the goals you have set for yourself. Slowly, you will find these daily activities becoming lifelong habits and helping you to overcome any obstacles standing in your way.

- **Review your goals regularly, and be willing to revise or abandon unreasonable goals.** Just setting a goal does not guarantee that you will achieve it. But, if you have followed all of the steps listed above, it will ensure that you will be moving steadily forward toward the articulated goal. Sometimes, as you work through your sub-goals, you will determine that the end goal no longer makes sense. Perhaps an event has occurred that no longer makes the goal a priority. Remember that goals represent the way you see your life from today's perspective. Monitor your progress as you go, and change your goals as your perspective changes.

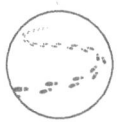

Action Steps

Gain Clarity About Your Current Physical Condition

- **Get A Physical**: Have you had a yearly physical that includes basic testing? Do you know your fasting glucose level? Lipid profile?
- Take a Health Assessment: Review your health history and concerns with a coach or other health practitioner to identify areas where you would like to implement changes so that you can work together to reach your goals.
- **Know Your Risk Factors for Heart Disease**: In addition to other tests used to assess heart problems, speak with your physician about having your Homocysteine and C-reactive protein levels tested. Another non-invasive procedure known as Intima-Media Thickness Scanning (IMT) is a safe and relatively inexpensive means of predicting the risk of heart attack or stroke.
- **Determine Your Risk For Diabetes**: Do you know your family history? If you have risk factors or symptoms, consult your physician to discuss testing.
- If You Have Diabetes, Know Your Numbers: Do you test your blood sugar levels regularly? Do you know your average blood sugar levels based on an HBA1C test?
- **Check Your Weight**: Is it within the range for your height and age? Do you know your muscle mass to fat ratio? What is your waist circumference?
- Check Your Blood Pressure: Is it within the normal range? If you don't know, make arrangements to have your blood pressure tested. If it is not within normal range, discuss treatment with your physician.

- **Check Your Exercise and Fitness Level**: Do you get some form of exercise at least once a day? If you don't currently have an exercise program, confirm that you don't have any conditions that would impede starting an exercise routine.
- **Review Your Medications**: Regarding any medications you may be taking, do you know the type, long-term effects, contraindications, alternatives, and the overall course of action recommended by your physician? If you have any questions or concerns, review them with your doctor.
- **Take Care of Your Eyes and Feet**: If diabetic, have you had your eyes and feet examined at least yearly? If not, schedule an appointment.
- Take Care of Your Kidneys: If diabetic, have you had your microalbumin levels measured? If not, discuss having this test performed with your physician.
- **If Symptomatic, Check for Thyroid Disease**: If you have any symptoms of thyroid disease, have you scheduled a TSH test? If the results were within normal range, have you discussed more in-depth testing with your physician in order to test the levels of the T4 and T3 thyroid hormones in your blood? Speak with your family physician or a specialist if your TSH test is within normal range, but your symptoms persist.

Gain Clarity About Your Food Consumption

To help you gain greater clarity about the foods you are eating, I created an assessment exercise designed to uncover eating behaviors that affect insulin resistance, blood sugar management, and living a sugar-free lifestyle. As you move through the remaining steps in the Roadmap, you can refer back to this exercise to identify habits holding you back and then make plans to put effective changes in place.

Have fun with this exercise. Do not "overthink" your responses. There are no right or wrong answers. You can't change a habit until you are fully conscious of the behavior. The main purpose of the exercise is to bring your habits to your full awareness and to get you thinking about what you eat on a daily basis.

- If you use colored pencils or pens to fill in the checkbox with the appropriate color, the resulting diagrams will provide you with a visual of where you are at the start of the challenge and the areas where you were able to make changes.

- (If you do not have colored pencils or pens, you can fill in the box by entering the letters G, Y, or R).
- There are 3 "columns" in the assessment. The First provides the item being assessed. The Second sets forth the optimal servings or other measurements suggested for the item. The Third guides you on how to rate your current behavior for each item.
- The time frame that you should use as applicable is current:
- (i.e., how you have been eating/living at the time of filling in the form --- over the last two to four weeks)
- Example: It is optimal to eat 1-2 servings of non-starchy vegetables with each meal. If you currently do this 5-7 days a week, either place the letter "G" in the "Non-Starchy Vegetable" checkbox or use a green pen or pencil to fill in the checkbox.

DATE OF ASSESSMENT:

	Item	Optimal Recommendation	Rating	Rating Description
Eat More	Non-starchy Vegetables	1-2 Servings each Meal/ Snack		**GREEN:** I consume 5-7 Days a week **YELLOW:** I eat occasionally. **RED:** I rarely consume
	Healthy Protein	1 Serving each Meal/ Snack		
	Healthy Fats	1 Serving each Meal/ Snack		
Avoid Or Eliminate	Added Sugar	Eliminate*		**GREEN:** I rarely consume **YELLOW:** I eat 3-5 times a week **RED:** I eat often or every day **Added sugar less than 1 gram OK on occasion,
	White Potatoes	Avoid		
	Grain-based flour products	Eliminate		
	Rice	White Rice (Eliminate)		
		Brown Rice (Avoid)		

Item	Optimal Recommendation	Rating	Rating Description
Soda	Regular Soda (Eliminate)		unless any added sugar is a trigger food.
	Diet Soda (Avoid)		
Fruit	High Glycemic (Eliminate)		
	Medium Glycemic (Avoid)		
	Low Glycemic (Consume Sparingly)		
Whole Grains	Quinoa (Consume Occasionally)		
	Other Grains (Avoid or consume in small portions occasionally		
Starchy Vegetables	Consume in small portions occasionally.		

Assess Your "Primary" Foods

The Lifestyle Assessment is designed to examine how balanced you are across different spheres of your physical, mental and spiritual life. It is a powerful tool because it gives you a vivid visual representation of the way your life is currently, compared with the way you would ideally like it to be. You can then use this assessment to identify areas that you would like to change and incorporate these into your vision, goals, and action plan. You can also revisit this assessment at various times to measure progress in different areas of your life.

This assessment is important in the context of going sugar-free to help you correlate the state of certain areas of your life to triggers that lead you to sugar consumption.

There are two ways you can use this tool. One way is to use the diagram with each segment pre-defined. Alternatively, you can create a personalized assessment by using a blank diagram and filling in the categories that are relevant to you.

This allows you to define your dimensions to fit your specific needs, priorities, and life experiences. Both options are available in this chapter. Examples of ways to personalize the Wheel can be by roles in life, such as husband/wife, father/mother, sports player, community leader, or friend. Another option is to personalize the Wheel by areas of life that are important to you, such as recovery, artistic expression, positive attitude, education, friends, spirituality, or public service. The key is to select areas of life that reflect your important priorities.

The center ring of the Wheel is 0, meaning you are dissatisfied with that aspect of life. The outer edge of the wheel is 10 and represents satisfaction and achievement with that aspect of your life.

Decide the degree of satisfaction from 0 to 10 and then mark it on the relevant spoke. When all areas have been marked, draw a line to connect the degree marks around the wheel. A graph appears that will give you a visual representation of how balanced your life is based on all the areas representing your life priorities.

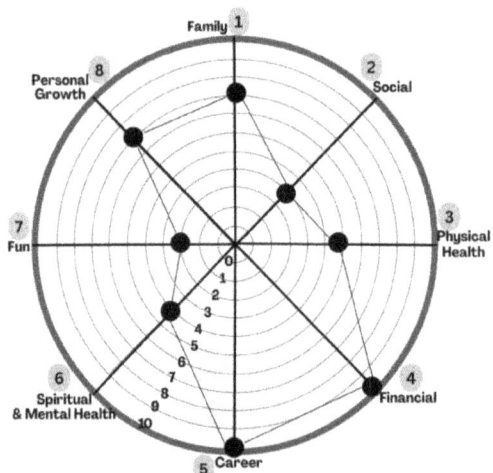

Lifestyle Assessment (Defined)

- Family/Relationship/Romance
- Community/Social/Friends
- Physical Health/Fitness
- Life Planning/Management/Financial Security/Money
- Career/Work/Vocation

- Spirituality/Morality
- Fun/Recreation/Leisure
- Personal Growth/Development/Learning

Rate each aspect on the Wheel from 0 to 10 and mark it on the relevant spoke. When all areas have been marked, draw a line connecting the degree marks around the wheel. The questions on the following page can assist with rating each aspect.

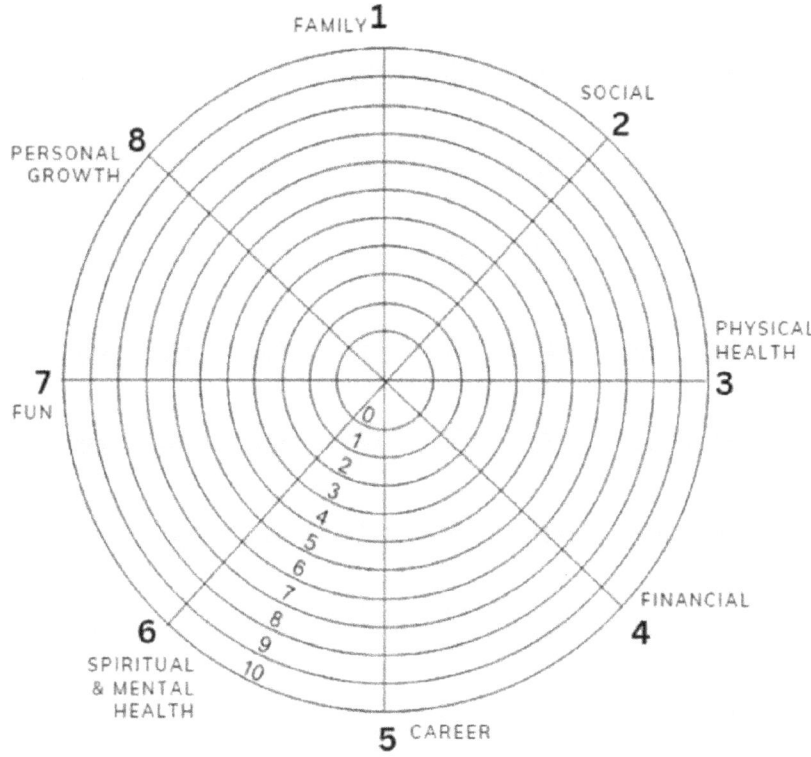

Lifestyle Assessment (Self-Defined)

List the Categories that are most significant to you, and use those for your Lifestyle Assessment.

1) _____

2) _____

3) _____

4) _____

5) _____

6) _____

7) _____

8) _____

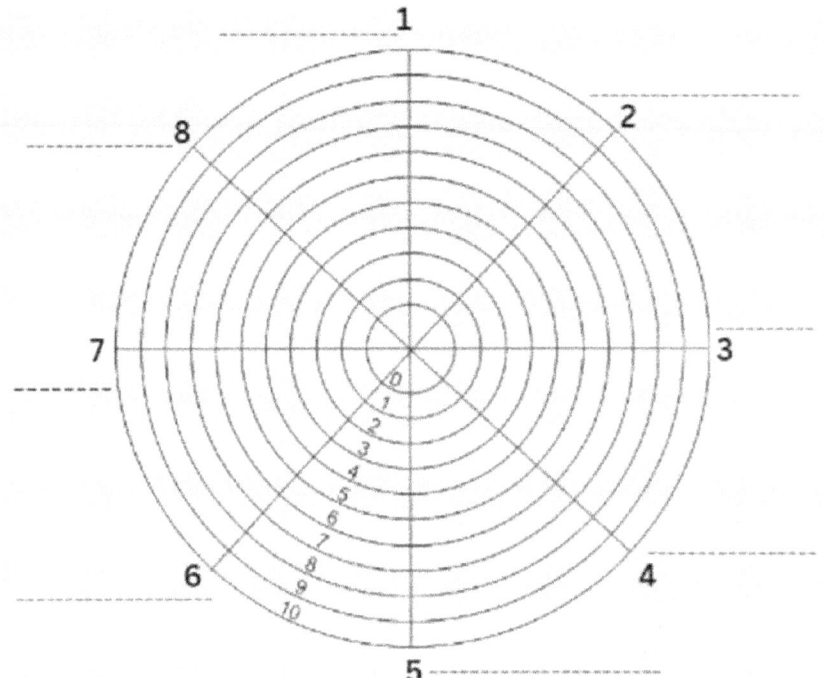

Questions to Aid in Completing Your Lifestyle Assessment

These questions are designed for your benefit and can help you better understand your current daily lifestyle. It can be helpful to write your responses in a journal and use your answers to guide you in determining how your life circumstances may be affecting your consumption of sugar and other trigger foods. Once you have more clarity about what you are eating daily and the areas of your life that you want to improve, you can develop your Vision and Goals that you want to achieve.

Can you begin to see how quitting sugar is more than following a food plan?

1. **Family/Relationship/Romance/Significant other**

- How content are you with your relationships with your family/significant other?
- How would you rate the quality of your home environment?

2. **Community/Social/Friends**

- How would you score the breadth and depth of friendships that you enjoy?
- Do you have time to socialize and make new friends and connections?
- Do you receive emotional support from friends and your community?

3. **Health/Wellbeing**

- How content are you with your eating habits, food plan, health, and fitness?
- Are you happy with the quality and quantity of your sleep?

4. **Life Planning/Management/Financial Security/Money**

- How financially secure do you feel?
- Are you able to set and keep to a budget?
- How free of debt are you?

5. **Career/Work/Vocation**

- How happy and fulfilled do you feel in your career or vocation?
- How content are you with the hours you work?
- Are you able to prioritize and manage your time?
- How content are you with your work prospects, progression, or promotion?

6. **Spiritual/Moral**

- Do you have an overall vision, purpose, and direction for your life?
- Do you spend time connecting with your internal self with activities such as personal reflection, prayer, or meditation?
- How happy are you with the legacy you are building and will leave behind?

7. **Fun/Recreation**

- Do you make time each week for leisure and recreation?
- Are you content with your ability to pursue your passions or hobbies?
- How energized do you feel?

8. **Personal Growth/Learning/Development**

- Are you content with the time you have for reading, listening, and learning?
- How self-aware would you say that you are?
- Are you content with your opportunity to develop existing strengths and learn new skills?

Assess Emotions that Impact Your Well-Being

Do any of the Feelings/Emotions in the chart below apply to you? Indicate the occurrence level by placing a checkmark in the columns corresponding to each emotion that applies to you in the table below.

Do your feelings track your answers in your Lifestyle Assessment? To increase positive emotions, what changes would you like to make? You can use the Vision and Goal Setting Exercises to create an action plan to implement any desired changes.

Feelings	Never	Rarely	Occasionally	Often	Every Day
Angry					
Anxious					
Depressed					
Deprived					
Nervous					
Sad					
Tired					
Worried					
Calm					

Feelings	Never	Rarely	Occasionally	Often	Every Day
Confident					
Energized					
Excited					
Hopeful					
Joyful					
Peaceful					
Proud					
Other:					

Create Your Vision

Develop your life vision using the worksheet below. You may not have all the answers right now. That's okay, take your time and add to it as you think of additional items.

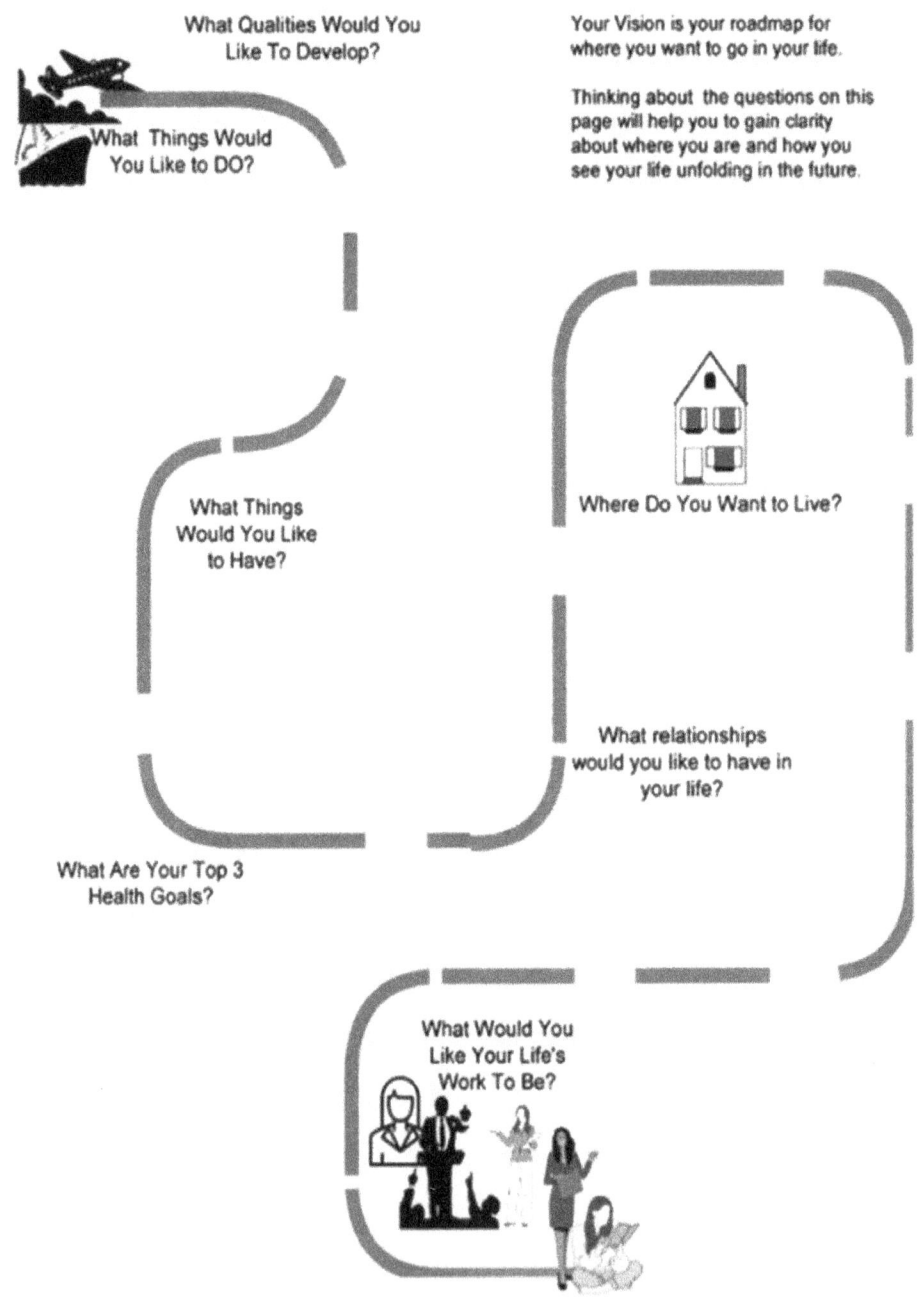

Additional Tips and Action Steps for Developing Your Vision

- Remember, good health is a state of complete physical, mental, social, and spiritual well-being, and not merely an absence of disease. Start brainstorming. How much would you like to weigh? What type of food plan would you like to incorporate into your lifestyle? What would you like to be doing 1 year, 5 years, 10 years from now?
- From this vision, you will be able to set concrete goals and communicate your vision to your medical care providers so that they can assist you in reaching your vision of health. If you are having trouble coming up with your vision statement, try the exercise on the preceding page as a starting point.

Write In Your Journal

- An effective technique when you are feeling stuck is to spend 5-10 minutes in the morning writing whatever comes to mind. There is no right or wrong way to write these thoughts in your journal. The point is to let your conscious mind go and let yourself express emotions and feelings that are holding you back. If you write faithfully in your journal first thing in the morning for a period of time, you will find a greater connection to the source of wisdom within you that will help you claim the life you want to lead.

Create a Vision Board

- If you are feeling stuck about creating your future vision, a vision board is a creative and fun way to get started. A vision board is a visual representation or collage of the things you want to have, be, or do in your life. Typically, it consists of a poster or foam board with cut-out pictures, drawings, and/or writing on it of the things that represent your desires, objectives, dreams, and goals. There are also companies that provide software programs so that you can create an electronic vision board. The purpose of creating a vision board is to start the process of attracting the events and circumstances into your life that will enable you to manifest your vision so that it becomes a reality.
- Your vision board can be very simple or complex. The key elements of a vision board are 1) a visual design that stimulates your mind, 2) pictures and words

that evoke a positive emotional response, and 3) location in a strategic place for maximum exposure.

Seek Assistance

- If journaling or other techniques are not sufficient, and you feel depressed or unable to make needed changes to improve your health, seek assistance from your primary physician or enlist assistance from other sources such as a counselor or diabetes coach.

In some cases, very powerful beliefs about ourselves developed over a lifetime can inhibit our ability to envision the life we desire. The book, "The Power of Belief," by Ray Dodd, explores these issues and provides a roadmap for identifying beliefs holding you back and for putting new beliefs in their place. This can be a good place to start if you feel stuck, and working through this process with a life coach can be helpful.

Create Short and Long Term Goals

Based on your Life Vision, identify your current goals using the timeframes described below. Then create sub-goals and supporting activities in the Creating Goals/Sub-Goals Exercise.

As your life circumstances change, revisit your goal plan and update it to add new goals, eliminate old ones, or reframe changed goals. I revisit my goal plan a few times each year.

	Short/Long Term Goals
1 Month Goals	
3 Month Goals	

Short/Long Term Goals
6 Month Goals
1 Year Goals
5 Year Goals
Lifetime Goals

Create Sub-Goals and Activities for Each High-Level Goal

Select one goal from your Short/Long Term Goals list, and use the Action Plan Worksheet below to create sub-goals and activities that will help you achieve this goal. Use the worksheet provided or a goal planning tool of your choice to create your action plan. I print out the Short/Long Term Goals and Action Plan worksheets and keep them in a binder so that I can keep them together and easily replace or update them as needed. (You can copy or print these worksheets from the Appendix or find digital downloads in our coaching community.)

When you are ready, repeat this exercise for each of your goals. If possible, include both a description of the goal/sub-goals as well as a time frame for starting and completing these goals. Goals, sub-goals, and timeframes may change as your life circumstances change. Be flexible and update your goals, sub-goals, and timeframes as needed.

Action Plan (Goal/Sub-Goals/Activities)	
GOAL	
Sub-Goal #1	
• SG#1 Activities	
• SG#1 Obstacles & Solutions	
Sub-Goal #2	
• SG#2 Activities	
• SG#2 Obstacles & Solutions	
Sub-Goal #3	
• SG#3 Activities	
• SG#3 Obstacles & Solutions	

Takeaways & Highlights

- The foundation for an effective action plan is having clarity about your vision for the future and the goals you want to achieve
- Clarity tools include guided support, assessments, journaling, meditation, and introspection.
- When you are having difficulties, your action plan is a tool you can rely on to reinforce positive lifestyle choices. When you find yourself going off-track, you can use your written action plan to get back to basics.

There are two aspects of your action plan:

- The pre-defined 3-phased Roadmap, including Action Steps specific to creating and maintaining a sugar-free lifestyle.
- The vision, goals, and related action steps are personal to you. These goals are the foundation of your "why" for going sugar-free and will differ for every participant in the Break Free from the Sugar Blues Program.

Vision and goal setting steps include the following:

- Develop your vision.
- Sketch out a plan.
- Translate your plan into written goals and sub-goals.
- Define activities and action steps.
- Identify obstacles and solutions.
- Establish reasonable deadlines for achieving your goals.
- Learn to distinguish goals from open-ended desires.
- Take daily, consistent action to achieve your goals
- Review your goals regularly, and be willing to revise or abandon unreasonable goals.

PHASE TWO:
Nourish Your Body to Live Free from Sugar

- Learn How Your Body Works: The Sugar, Mind, and Body Connection
- Implement a Food Plan that Eliminates Personal Trigger Foods
- Validate, Monitor, and Adjust Your Plan
- Enhance Your Food Plan with Exercise, Restful Sleep, and Stress Management

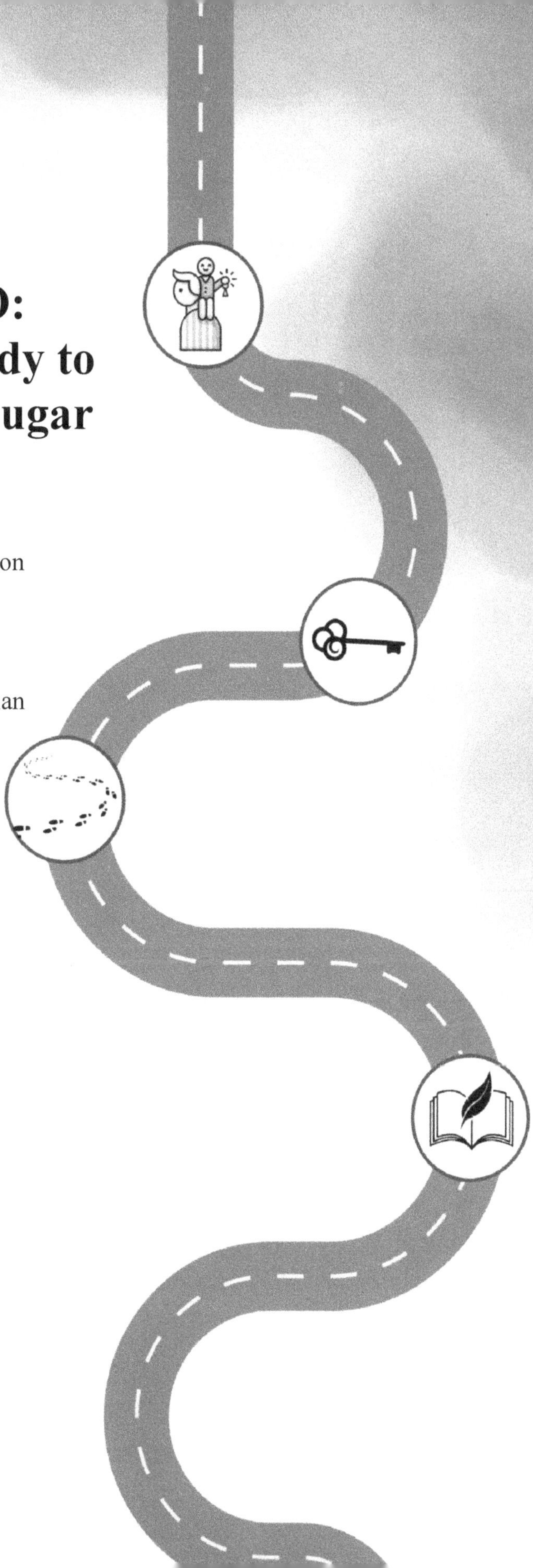

CHAPTER 11
Learn How Your Body Works: The Sugar, Mind, and Body Connection

Coach on Your Shoulder

Information is Empowerment

The purpose of this chapter is to teach you how your body works so that you can control what and how you eat. When you understand how sugar and other carbohydrates are digested, you will gain the knowledge and confidence to make food choices that are right for you.

I know it is tempting to skip this chapter and go straight to the food plan. Most people have been led to believe it's too hard to understand how their body works, especially how different foods affect their health. Figuring out what to eat is quite a dilemma for both young and old.

We want experts to give us the answers. Who cares how our body works, right? We can leave that stuff to the doctors and nutritionists. You are probably thinking, "Isn't that why I bought this book? Can't you, the expert, tell me what to eat?" Unfortunately, diets consisting of a restrictive set of instructions with pre-ordained boundaries (usually points, calories, amount of carbohydrates, or some other type of measurement) seem easy to follow at the outset. However, over time, the same limitations that attract most people to the program end up being impossible to follow in the long term.

You can be assured that this book provides a comprehensive food plan with a list of recommended foods and guidelines optimal for a sugar-free lifestyle. It also provides you with all the information you need to make food choices that are right for you. However, the food plan is not a rigid set of must-follow rules. It goes beyond the typical diet approach by providing you with a set of guidelines, plus the knowledge and guidance that support your ability to make decisions based on a range of options while learning to make decisions that empower you to eat in a way that:

- Works in harmony with your unique biochemistry,
- Keeps your blood sugar and insulin levels in a balanced state,
- Eliminates your personal trigger foods,
- Conquers cravings, and
- Helps you to stick with it for the long term.

The good news is that you don't need to become a medical expert to understand the relationship between sugar and how it affects your body.

Think of it this way. There is a saying: "Give a man a fish, and you feed him for a day. Teach him how to fish, and you feed him for a lifetime."

Likewise, you can go on a quick fix "diet" that skips the self-knowledge part and typically lasts until frustration sets in or willpower fails. A different option is to connect with your body and gain the confidence that empowers you to make daily decisions that move you toward your goals and help you stay on track.

By the end of this chapter, you will no longer be controlled by a set of external rules. Instead, you will understand how different carbohydrates function in your body, and you will have greater insight into which foods to include in your food plan and which foods to avoid. If you are working with a nutritionist or food coach, you will know what questions to ask and how to leverage their support to make decisions that work for you.

Key Concepts

Carbohydrates, Digestion, and Blood Sugar Levels

Of all the foods in your plan, the amount and type of carbohydrates you consume will have the most significant impact on your blood sugar levels and unwanted effects, such as cravings and weight gain.

Understanding how carbohydrates work in your body will help you make choices that support normal blood sugar levels.

Let's start by taking a 1000-foot view of what happens when you eat sugar and other carbohydrates. Then, we will zoom in to learn about the different types of carbohydrates and how carbohydrates affect your body. We will also take a more detailed view of how hormones such as insulin and glucagon work in your body to balance your blood sugar levels and turn food into energy.

Think of your body as a huge chemical processing plant designed to provide your cells with energy so that you can function. As described below, your body is an amazing symphony of coordinated processes designed to keep your blood sugar levels and associated bodily functions balanced.

- The fuel of choice for cells is the simple sugar glucose, and carbohydrates are the primary food source for glucose.
- When you eat added sugar and other carbohydrates, your body ultimately breaks down the carbohydrates into glucose and/or another type of simple sugar called fructose, depending on the type of carbohydrate eaten. Each of these simple sugars passes into your bloodstream for further processing.
- When glucose enters your bloodstream, your blood sugar levels begin to rise, prompting your body to release insulin.
- In turn, insulin triggers your cells to take up the glucose to use for generating energy (or to store it for later use) and to return blood sugar levels to normal.

What are Carbohydrates Made Of?

- Carbohydrates are not foods but rather collections of molecules consisting of carbon, oxygen, and hydrogen.
- Chemically, at their most basic level, ALL carbohydrates are made up of units of sugar. These sugar units are called saccharide units.
- Physically, carbohydrates take the form of sugars, starches, and cellulose.
- There are two main classifications of carbohydrates: simple sugars and complex carbohydrates. Starches and cellulose are two types of complex carbohydrates.
- Some complex carbohydrates, like potatoes, act more like simple carbohydrates in your system, and the amount of processed foods consumed also has a significant impact on how carbohydrates affect your blood sugars.

As you will learn in the next section, simple sugars are broken down quickly to release energy and enter the bloodstream more rapidly, causing a fast rise in blood glucose accompanied by a sharp rise in insulin. Most complex carbohydrates are digested more slowly and moderate the glucose and insulin response, but there are exceptions. Foods such as white potatoes, rice, or whole grain flour can be tricky because they digest more like a simple sugar.

How Carbohydrates are Classified

Below is a chart, introduced in Chapter 9, that provides an overview of the different types of carbohydrates classified as simple sugars and complex carbohydrates, which are also further grouped by their chemical makeup as monosaccharides, disaccharides, oligosaccharides, and polysaccharides. The latter groupings are based upon the number of sugar units present in the simple sugar or complex carbohydrate.

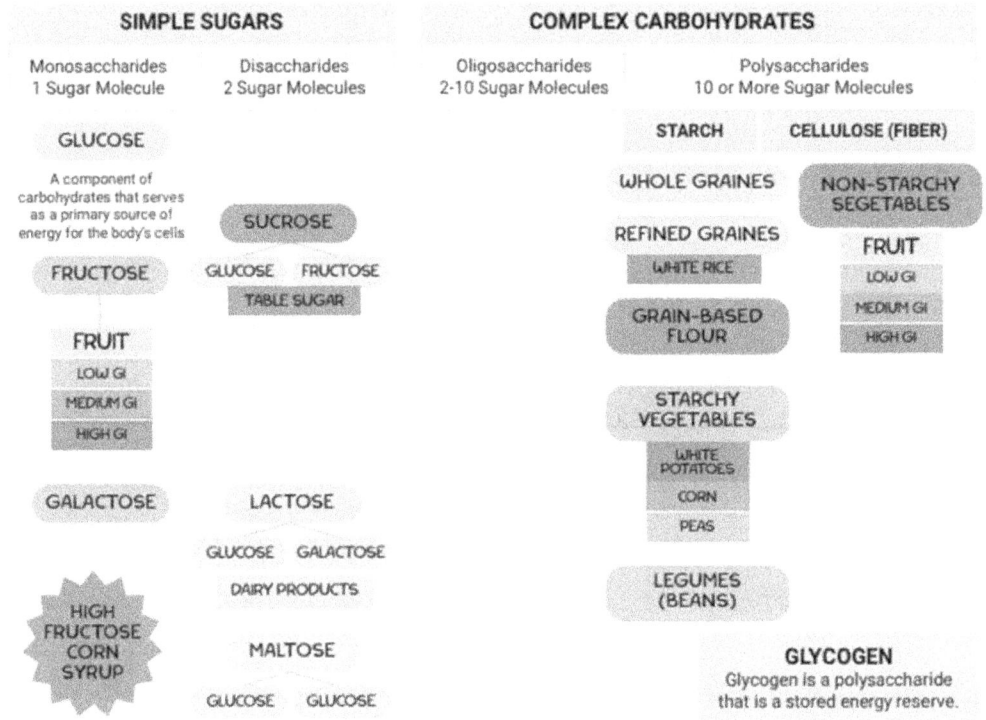

Types of Simple Sugars

Carbohydrates containing only one or two sugar units are called simple sugars. Simple sugars are often named according to the foodstuff with which they are associated, i.e., lactose (milk), maltose (malt, grain), fructose (fruit), and sucrose (refined sugar).

Simple sugars taste sweet and are broken down quickly in the body to release energy. This means they enter the bloodstream more rapidly causing a fast rise in blood glucose accompanied by a sharp rise in insulin to contain them. Fructose is a simple sugar, twice as sweet as sucrose (table sugar). Because it is mainly metabolized in the liver, fructose has a lower glycemic index. However, fructose is incorporated into triglycerides more readily than glucose (blood sugar); therefore, it has a greater propensity to increase serum triglycerides.

Monosaccharides are the simplest form of sugar and the most basic unit from which all carbohydrates are built. Only monosaccharides can be absorbed from the digestive tract into the blood, and in order to be used by our body as energy, all carbohydrate foods must first be digested into their monosaccharide subunits: glucose, fructose, or galactose.

Disaccharides are formed when two monosaccharide molecules are linked together. Disaccharides that are found in carbohydrate foods include sucrose, lactose and maltose. There are specific enzymes that break down disaccharides into monosaccharides: sucrase (to digest sucrose), lactase (to digest lactose), and maltase to digest maltose.

- **Sucrose** is often known as table sugar and is composed of two monosaccharides: glucose + fructose. Sucrose is found naturally in plants such as fruits, vegetables, and nuts. Sucrose is also commercially produced from sugar cane and sugar beets.
- **Lactose** is found in dairy foods and is composed of two monosaccharides: glucose + galactose.
- **Maltose** is found naturally in foods such as grains, cereals, molasses, and cooked sweet potatoes. Maltose is also used to sweeten beer during the manufacturing process, and it is also used as a sweetener in processed foods. Maltose is composed of two glucose units joined together.

Types of Complex Carbohydrates

Complex carbohydrates are long chains of simple sugar units bonded together. As a general rule, complex carbohydrates are digested more slowly and moderate the glucose and insulin response. Starch and cellulose are two types of complex carbohydrates.

Starch is a type of complex carbohydrate found in foods like potatoes, rice, and grains.

- Plants store starch in seeds or other specialized organs, where it remains until needed for energy, during periods of growth, or when photosynthesis is not possible.
- For example, starch in seeds gives the seedling energy to sprout, and we eat those seeds in the form of grains, legumes, nuts, and seeds.

- Starch is also stored in roots and tubers to provide stored energy for the plant to grow and reproduce, and we eat these in the form of potatoes, sweet potatoes, carrots, beets, and turnips.
- Starch from whole plant foods comes packaged with other valuable nutrients and fiber, and during the digestion process, starch is broken into soluble glucose units.

Foods such as white potatoes, rice, grains, and whole grain flour, despite being complex carbohydrates, are often digested more like simple sugars.

- The molecular structure of starches in these foods includes amylose and amylopectin, with amylopectin having a branched structure that is more easily broken down by digestive enzymes.
- When these foods are processed or cooked, their starches, particularly amylopectin, break down more rapidly, leading to a quick spike in blood sugar.
- This rapid digestion can cause a surge of energy followed by a sudden drop, similar to the effects of consuming simple sugars. Consequently, while these foods are generally healthier than pure, simple sugars, their impact on blood sugar levels requires mindful consumption.

Cellulose differs from the complex carbohydrate starch because its glucose units form a two-dimensional structure, giving the molecule added stability.

- Also known as plant or dietary fiber, cellulose cannot be digested by human beings. (It passes through the digestive tract without being broken down by human digestive enzymes.)
- Cellulose is a relatively stiff material, and in plants, it serves as a structural molecule to provide support to the leaves, stem, and other plant parts.
- Although it cannot be used as an energy source in most animals, cellulose fiber is essential in the diet because it helps exercise the digestive tract and keeps it clean and healthy.
- Additionally, fiber slows digestion, which has a beneficial effect on blood sugar levels.

Polysaccharides are long chains of monosaccharide subunits linked together and are what we refer to as complex carbohydrates. These chains may number from as few as three subunits to thousands. Based on their function, polysaccharides can be classified as either storage molecules or structural molecules.

- Storage polysaccharides include two types: starch and glycogen.
- Starch is the storage form of carbohydrates in plants. Starch sources include seeds, grains, corn, beans, potatoes, and rice.
- Glycogen is the storage form of carbohydrate in animals. We store glycogen primarily in our livers and skeletal muscles. The glycogen in skeletal muscle can be depleted with as little as 1 hour of vigorous exercise. On the other hand, during a fast, liver glycogen will last 12-24 hours. That shaky feeling you get at the end of a fast is largely due to a depletion of your glycogen stores.
- Cellulose is a structural polysaccharide.
- Cellulose forms the structural components of plant cell walls and provides the fiber you need in your diet. However, unlike starches and glycogen, humans do not have the enzymes to digest cellulose for energy use. Fiber, along with protein and fats, helps to slow down the digestion of carbohydrates and delay their absorption into the blood. This helps to prevent spikes in glucose levels after eating.

Oligosaccharides are also long chains of monosaccharide subunits linked together, but they are made up of 2 to 10 simple sugars.

- Oligosaccharides are found in certain vegetables, fruits, grains, and legumes.
- The human digestive tract cannot break down the large majority of oligosaccharides. Instead, they travel through your gut to the colon, where they feed and support the growth of beneficial bacteria.
- Because of this, oligosaccharides are considered prebiotics, and their prebiotic properties offer many health benefits, including improved digestion and gut health

The 3 Metabolic States

The rise and fall of your blood sugar levels is a natural part of your body's metabolism following a meal, and your daily eating patterns affect the availability of glucose for your body to use as energy. Most of us eat periodically throughout the day and sometimes into the evening. Sometimes, you eat continuously (such as when you eat a meal and have a snack within a few hours), and at other times, you might go for longer periods without eating.

Your organs, especially the brain, need a continuous supply of glucose to function properly. To meet this constant energy demand, your body processes food through mechanisms that allow some of the food to be broken down into glucose and used immediately for energy, while also storing some of the glucose in your liver and muscles for later use. If these mechanisms did not exist to store energy, you would have to eat constantly to meet your body's energy needs.

This is why the Sugar-Free Lifestyle Food Plan™ is based on the principle of eating in harmony with how your body works. As you will learn, when you eat foods that support balanced blood sugar levels, you can avoid insulin resistance, cravings, yo-yo weight gain, and other blood sugar health issues. When you consistently eat added sugar and other foods that cause sharp/fast blood sugar spikes, things tend to go awry.

The mechanisms that facilitate both immediate energy use and energy storage occur within three metabolic states.

- Postprandial or Absorptive State
- Post Absorptive or Fasting State
- Prolonged Fasting State

These three metabolic states are characterized by:

- When they occur,
- How long they last,
- The metabolic activity that occurs in each, and
- The hormones produced to facilitate the metabolic activity in each state.

Keep in mind that you move in and out of these metabolic states several times in a 24-hour period based on the type of food you eat, the timing of consumption, blood glucose concentration, and hormonal responses to the changes occurring throughout the digestion process. There are general guidelines that describe the amount of time that each metabolic state lasts, but the exact timing of these transitions will depend upon your unique biochemistry and state of health.

The diagram below provides an overview of the processes that occur in the three metabolic states.

Metabolic States Overview

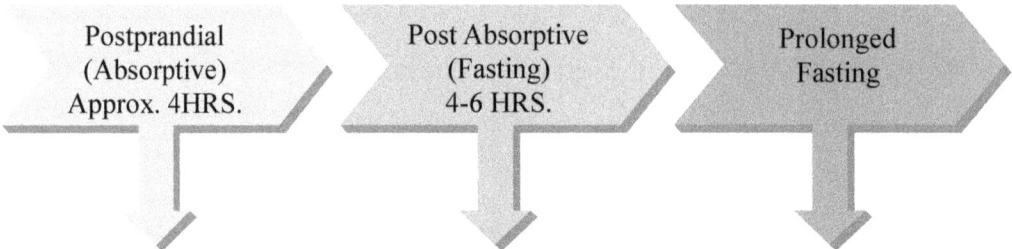

Postprandial (Absorptive) Approx. 4HRS. →	Post Absorptive (Fasting) 4-6 HRS. →	Prolonged Fasting →
Food is Digested and Nutrients Absorbed	**Glycogen is Utilized to Keep Blood Sugar Levels Stable**	**Blood Glucose Levels Fall**
Carbohydrates are chewed, swallowed, and processed into chyme in the stomach. The chyme enters the small intestine, where enzymes break down carbohydrates into glucose, fructose, and galactose.

Glucose enters the bloodstream, and blood sugar levels rise.

Beta cells in the pancreas produce insulin, which stimulates the cells' uptake of glucose for immediate energy. A portion of glucose is stored in skeletal muscles and the liver as glycogen for later use. Excess glucose is stored as fat.

Blood sugar levels begin to fall, initiating the Post Absorptive (Fasting) State. | This metabolic state lasts for approximately 4-6 hours following the postprandial state. (Assuming that no new nutrients have been eaten. If yes, you are back in Postprandial)

Typically, glucose levels continue to fall. If glucose levels in the bloodstream begin to fall below normal levels, alpha cells in the pancreas start producing glucagon, a hormone that stimulates the breakdown of stored glycogen in the liver and skeletal muscles, converting it back into glucose.

If glucose levels begin to rise, insulin promotes glucose absorption by cells & any excess is stored as fat. | The effects of prolonged fasting kick in 10-12 hours after your last food has been consumed.

If there is not enough glucose available to provide energy during prolonged fasting, the body adopts an alternative strategy to meet these needs. Specifically, it begins to break down fat stores, allowing them to be used as an energy source.

This process involves the breakdown of stored triglycerides within fat cells (adipocytes) and the subsequent utilization of fatty acids as an energy source. |

The Postprandial Metabolic State

Postprandial Process: The Roles of Glucose and Insulin

The first metabolic state, *Postprandial*, begins as soon as you start eating and lasts approximately 4 hours. As described below, after your food is broken down into its basic components, glucose is released into your bloodstream, and your pancreas releases insulin to stimulate the uptake of glucose by your cells to be used as energy.

Postprandial Process Overview	Description
1. Digestion Starts When You Eat, Chew & Swallow Food	• The first step in digestion is breaking food down into smaller particles so the food can move through the esophagus to your stomach • During the chewing process, food is also mixed with salivary enzymes needed for digestion.
2. Food Is Processed Into Its Basic Elements	• After food has been processed in your stomach, the chyme (what food is now called) passes into the first part of the small intestine, where enzymes break down proteins into amino acids and fats into fatty acids. • Carbohydrates are ultimately broken down into their simplest form: glucose, fructose, or galactose.
3. Glucose is Released Into the Bloodstream & Blood Glucose Levels Rise	• The amount of glucose that enters the bloodstream and how fast blood sugar levels rise impact how much insulin is released to transport a portion of glucose out of your bloodstream.
4. The Pancreas Beta Cells Produce Insulin to Move Glucose Into Cells for Immediate Energy or Into Storage for Later Use	• Insulin moves a portion of the glucose in your bloodstream into your cells to be used as an immediate energy source, or it moves a portion into your muscles and liver, where it is stored as a substance called glycogen for later use.
5. Blood Sugar Levels Fall	• As cells absorbed glucose, blood sugar levels begin to fall, initiating the next metabolic state: Post Absorptive/Fasting.

Postprandial Process: Chewing and Swallowing

Your body uses two methods to break down food: chemical and mechanical digestion. Mechanical digestion involves physical movement to break food down into smaller particles. Chemical digestion uses enzymes to break the chemical bonds that hold food particles together. The combination of mechanical and chemical digestion allows food to be broken down into small, digestible parts.

When you take a bite of food, mechanical digestion begins with the physical act of chewing, which physically breaks down the food into smaller particles. During the chewing process, food is broken down into smaller particles, and salivary glands in the mouth release enzymes, including salivary amylase and lingual lipase.

Salivary amylase begins the chemical breakdown of complex carbohydrates (starches) into sugars that are more easily absorbed. Saliva also contains an enzyme called lingual lipase, which breaks down fats. When we are done chewing, we swallow the smaller, more digestible food particles, which then move through the esophagus to the stomach. The stomach's primary tool for digestion is the potent mix of secretions collectively called gastric juices, which process the food into a highly acidic mixture known as chyme.

Although starch digestion begins in the mouth, the majority of carbohydrate digestion occurs in the small intestine, where enzymes are released during the chemical digestion process.

Postprandial Process: The Breakdown of Carbohydrates

After the muscular and chemical actions of the stomach process food, the chyme passes into the first part of the small intestine. In the small intestine, the chyme is mixed with enzymes from the pancreas and bile from the liver/gallbladder. These enzymes further the process of digestion by breaking down proteins, fat, and carbohydrates.

Carbohydrates are broken down both mechanically (e.g., through chewing) and chemically (e.g., by enzymes) into the single units glucose, fructose, and/or galactose. These are absorbed into the bloodstream and distributed throughout the body to be used as energy or stored as fat.

The way in which different types of carbohydrates are digested has a major impact on blood sugar levels and our overall health. In the next chapter, you are going to begin to create a food plan that will guide your food choices on a daily basis. Of all the foods in your plan, the amount and type of carbohydrates that you eat will have the most dramatic impact on your blood sugar levels, and understanding how carbohydrates work in your body will help you to make choices that eliminate trigger foods and keep cravings at bay.

Postprandial Process: Glucose is Released into the Bloodstream, and Glucose Levels Rise

Once food is processed in the small intestine and carbohydrates have been converted into glucose, the glucose is absorbed and actively transported through the intestinal walls into the bloodstream, where it is available as a source of energy.

Choosing to eat (or reject) a food based on the amount of carbohydrates it contains only gives you a small piece of the carbohydrate puzzle. In order to successfully manage blood sugars, several factors should be considered, including type, processing, amount of carbohydrates consumed and the food's effect on blood sugar levels.

When you eat foods that cause a fast/sharp rise in glucose, we refer to this as a blood glucose spike. The amount of glucose and how fast it enters your bloodstream depends on a number of factors, including:

- **The type of carbohydrate eaten**: As a general rule, complex carbohydrates in their whole food form are processed more slowly, causing a more gradual increase in blood sugar. In contrast, foods that are high in simple carbohydrates are quickly digested and absorbed, leading to rapid spikes in blood sugar. Not all complex carbohydrates behave the way you expect them to. For example, starchy vegetables, like white potatoes, behave more like simple sugars, breaking down quickly into glucose, leading to a faster rise in blood glucose levels.
- **Portion size**: Larger portions can result in higher glucose levels because more carbohydrates are consumed at one time. Managing portion sizes can be a direct and effective method for controlling blood sugar levels.

- **The level of processing**: Refined carbohydrates are carbohydrates that have gone through a process that separates them from the minerals, vitamins, protein, and fiber that originally were present as co-worker nutrients that assist our bodies in metabolizing them. Like simple sugars, refined carbohydrates are digested very quickly, causing a fast rise in blood glucose, and for that reason, you should think of them as a hidden source of sugar in your diet.
- **Meal/snack composition**: The presence of fiber, fats, and proteins in a food, meal, or snack can also modulate blood sugar levels. Fiber, fats, and proteins slow the absorption of carbohydrates, resulting in more stable blood sugar levels. Choosing foods that are higher in fiber content, along with including healthy fats and proteins with meals and snacks, is an effective strategy to manage postprandial spikes.
- **The type of starch in the food**: There are two types of starch: amylose and amylopectin. It is the proportion of each form of starch in a particular food that determines the food's ability to be digested. Foods with a large amount of amylopectin are digested and absorbed rapidly, while foods that have higher levels of amylose break down at a slower rate.
- **Physical activity**: Activity level both before and after a meal can influence how the body processes glucose. Exercise helps muscles absorb glucose more effectively, reducing blood sugar spikes.
- **Your state of health and unique biochemistry**: Many things can affect how glucose is processed in your body, including insulin resistance, diabetes, weight, muscle mass, and mental state.

Postprandial Process: The Pancreas Produces Insulin to Move Glucose Out of the Bloodstream and Into Cells for Immediate Energy Use or Storage for Later Use

The pancreas is a large gland that is located in the abdomen, behind your stomach. The main function of the pancreas is to produce insulin, digestive enzymes, and other hormones that coordinate different functions in your body by carrying messages through your blood to your organs, skin, muscles, and other tissues. These signals tell your body what to do and when to do it.

- After you eat, digest, and absorb carbohydrate foods, your blood glucose level rises, and your body prepares to receive the glucose, fatty acids, and amino acids that have been absorbed from the food.
- In response to glucose entering our bloodstream, insulin is released from the pancreas, facilitating the uptake of glucose by tissues for use as energy and its storage as glycogen in the liver and muscles.
- The presence of these substances in the intestine stimulates the pancreatic beta cells to release insulin into the blood (and also inhibits the pancreatic alpha cells from secreting another hormone called glucagon). The amount of insulin released is directly proportional to how fast glucose levels rise and the amount of glucose entering the bloodstream.
- The levels of insulin in the blood begin to rise, and the release of insulin into the bloodstream facilitates the ability of cells to absorb the incoming molecules of glucose. Some cells use glucose immediately as energy. Other cells in your liver and muscles store any excess glucose as a substance called glycogen, which is held in reserve to be used for fuel when your body needs it, such as between meals.

Insulin acts as a "key," essentially unlocking tiny doors on cell walls (called insulin receptor sites) that allow glucose to enter the cells. As part of this process, insulin activates the production of glucose transporters within the cells. These specialized protein molecules emerge from the nuclei of the cells to grab glucose from the blood and bring it to the interiors of the cells. Once inside the cell, glucose can be utilized as an immediate power source to provide fuel for energy-requiring functions.

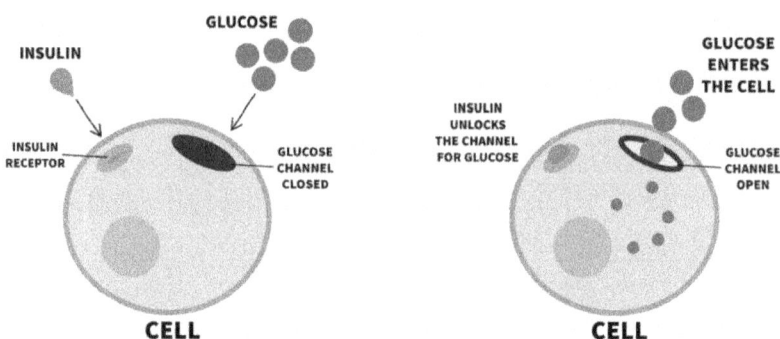

If there is more glucose in the bloodstream than is immediately needed for energy, insulin stimulates the liver and muscle cells to store this glucose in the form of glycogen for use when it is needed at a later time. The ultimate effect is that the action of insulin prevents the blood glucose concentration from substantially increasing in the bloodstream, and as insulin promotes the uptake of glucose by our cells, the amount of insulin in the bloodstream decreases.

The mechanism that stores excess glucose as glycogen helps to keep blood sugar levels normalized. You might think this is excellent, I can eat as much sugar as I want and never have to worry about sugar intake. But not so fast. The problem is that the ability of liver and muscle cells to store glycogen is not infinite, and when these cells reach their limit, another metabolic pathway opens up, leading to glucose being stored as fat.

Excess glucose is turned into fat through a chemical process called lipogenesis. When the body's glycogen storage capacities in the liver are saturated, insulin triggers a process called lipogenesis, where excess glucose is converted into fatty acids. These fatty acids are then assembled into triglycerides and stored in adipose (fat) tissue. This mechanism ensures that excess glucose is effectively removed from the bloodstream, but as we will learn at the end of this chapter, this fat storage brings on problems of its own.

When blood sugar levels start to fall, the next metabolic state, called postabsorptive or fasting, begins. During this state, another hormone, glucagon, is released by the alpha cells of the pancreas to instruct the liver and muscles to convert stored glycogen into glucose.

The release of glucagon ensures that your body's metabolic needs are met during periods when you are not consuming food so that the amount of glucose circulating in your bloodstream remains at a sufficient level to supply the brain and other glucose-dependent tissues with the glucose needed for energy. Maintaining normal blood sugar levels is essential to prevent hypoglycemia (low blood sugar), which can cause symptoms like dizziness, confusion, and even loss of consciousness. If your body is functioning normally, the levels of insulin and glucagon are counter-balanced to maintain overall metabolic balance as described in the next section.

Postabsorptive Metabolic State

Maintaining Balanced Blood Glucose Levels

The postabsorptive state begins when all of the processes in the postprandial state have ended and blood glucose levels are falling. This state lasts 10-12 hours and is also called the fasting state because during this time, the body isn't processing any nutrients from a meal or snack. Typically, your body goes into a postabsorptive state overnight, but skipping meals during the day (with no snacks in-between meals) can also put your body into a postabsorptive state.

As blood glucose levels begin to drop to below normal levels, glucagon is released to stimulate the conversion of stored glycogen back into glucose. This helps maintain blood glucose levels within a normal range.

How does your body know when to secrete glucagon or insulin?

If your body is functioning normally, the levels of insulin and glucagon are counter-balanced in the bloodstream in the following way:

When blood glucose levels rise, beta cells in the pancreas produce insulin to transport glucose into the cells, where it is used as energy or stored as glycogen for later use. If there is too much glucose on a regular basis, it will be stored as fat.

The insulin levels in your blood begin to rise, and the release of insulin into the bloodstream facilitates the ability of cells (particularly liver, fat, and muscle cells) to absorb the incoming molecules of glucose, fatty acids, and amino acids. As part of this process, insulin removes glucose from your bloodstream and brings it into the interior of your cells, where it can be utilized as an immediate power source to provide fuel for energy-requiring functions.

In contrast, when you are between meals or sleeping, glucose levels are typically falling, but your cells still need supplies of glucose from the blood in order to keep going.

During these times, slight drops in blood sugar levels stimulate glucagon secretion from the pancreatic alpha cells and inhibit insulin secretion from the beta cells.

As glucagon levels rise, glucagon acts on liver and muscle tissue to initiate a process whereby the glucagon "instructs" the liver and muscles to begin converting glycogen to glucose, which will be released into the bloodstream. This action prevents levels of glucose in your blood from falling drastically.

INSULIN:	GLUCAGON:
Is produced by the BETA cells of the pancreas	Is produced by the ALPHA cells of the pancreas
Is released when you have just eaten, and the level of glucose in your bloodstream is high.	Is released when your blood sugar levels are low (for example, if you have been fasting or exercising).
Stimulates the cells within your body to take up the glucose in your blood to be used either for immediate energy or for storing (as glycogen, a starchy substance stored both in the liver and muscle cells).	Stimulates the liver and muscles to break down stored glycogen and release the glucose into the bloodstream for use as energy.
When you have an oversupply of glucose in your bloodstream, your body stores the excess in the liver and muscles as glycogen. If there is too much glucose to store in your muscle cells or liver, it stores it as fat.	When glucose is in short supply, your body mobilizes glucose from stored glycogen and/or stimulates you to eat food.

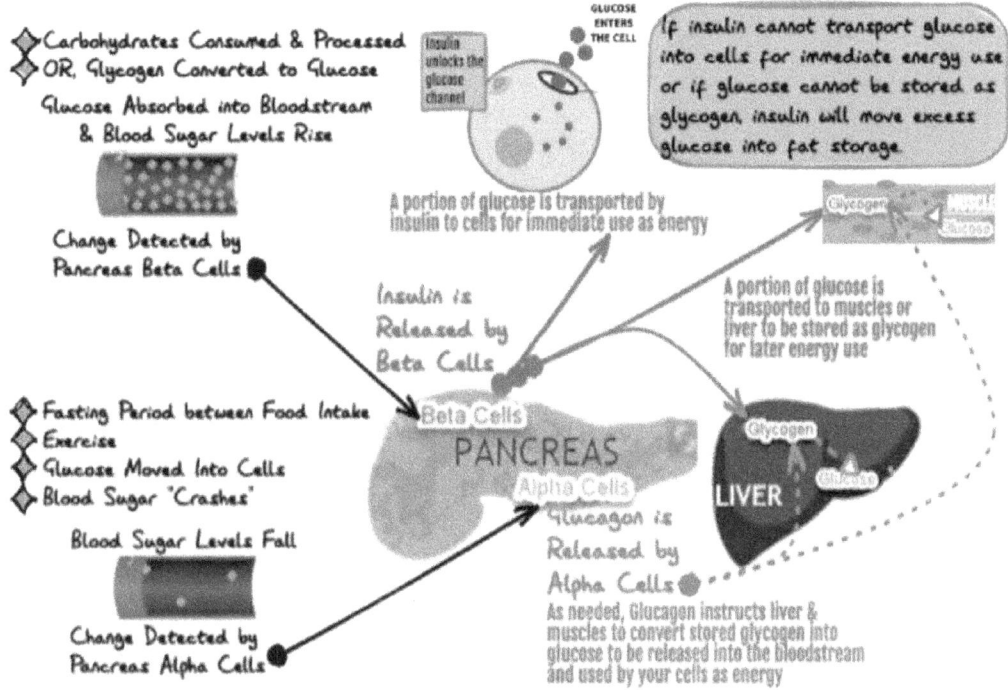

The Prolonged Fasting Metabolic State: Fat Burning

After the postabsorptive period (about 10-12 hours after eating), your body is in a fasted state until your next meal. In this phase, glycogen stores are depleted, and the body increasingly relies on fat as a primary energy source. This results in the breakdown of fat stores into fatty acids and glycerol, which are used directly for energy or converted into ketone bodies when fatty acid levels are high. This is why intermittent fasting can help with weight loss. It is achieved by setting an eating schedule that allows people to go more than 12 hours without eating, enabling their body to burn fat as its primary energy source for a period of time.

The problem for many people is that they are constantly eating, and so their body never gets the benefits of a fasted state where their body has a chance to burn fat. Additionally, if the foods they are eating cause constant glucose spikes and crashes, they may be storing excess glucose as fat, resulting in a double whammy: more fat storage and less fat burning.

Blood Sugar Spikes, Cravings and Insulin Resistance

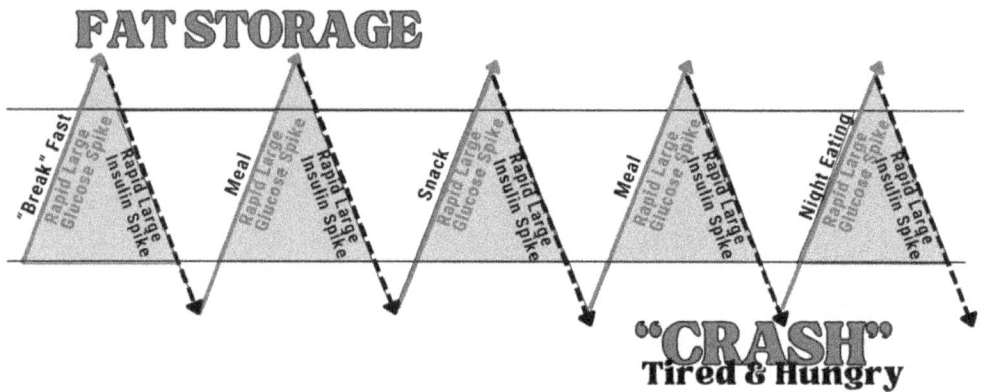

When we eat foods that cause a fast/sharp rise in glucose, we refer to this as a blood glucose spike. As they say, "what goes up, must come down," and what happens next is that insulin responds with enough insulin to carry the high levels of glucose out of our bloodstream, very often leading to low blood sugar levels or "crashes."

Eating added sugar or other foods that cause a fast/sharp rise in glucose infrequently does not cause a problem for most people. But if you consistently eat meals and snacks that cause blood sugar levels to rise quickly, your body can stay in a state of elevated blood glucose levels, requiring the body to regularly release insulin. This eating pattern can lead to roller-coaster blood sugar levels, along with insulin resistance and the storage of excess glucose as fat.

On the surface, it seems that having excess insulin is a good thing. You might think that if we have more insulin than we need, we will always have enough to keep our blood sugar under control, and hence we won't get diabetes or have other problems. But it is just the opposite.

The life-promoting qualities of insulin can be a double-edged sword when there is too much glucose or too much insulin in the bloodstream on a habitual basis. Few people realize that once glycogen storage sites in the muscles and liver are filled, excess glucose remaining in the bloodstream is converted to and stored as fat. This is just one of the consequences of habitual high blood sugar levels.

When people are insulin resistant, their muscle, fat, and liver cells do not respond properly to insulin. As a result, their bodies need more insulin to help glucose enter cells. The pancreas tries to keep up with this increased demand for insulin by producing more. Eventually, the pancreas fails to keep up with the body's need for insulin. Excess glucose builds up in the bloodstream, setting the stage for pre-diabetes and full-blown diabetes. Many people with insulin resistance have high levels of both glucose and insulin circulating in their blood at the same time.

On the following pages, we will explore what happens when the system breaks down and the body can no longer maintain the delicate balancing act that keeps our blood sugars in a normal range.

Insulin and Fat Storage

Few people realize that in addition to helping to regulate blood sugar levels, insulin also helps to store fat.

You have learned that after you eat, digest, and absorb carbohydrate foods, your blood sugar level normally rises. Then, the pancreas responds by releasing insulin, which transports the glucose into your cells where it can be used as energy.

Most people are surprised to learn that when you have more glucose in your body than your cells need, insulin takes the extra glucose and transports it into fat storage. This is, in one sense, a good thing because it helps (at least in the short term) to prevent high levels of glucose from remaining in the bloodstream. However, when insulin levels rise and spike in an effort to control high blood sugar levels, more fat is also stored.

Visceral Obesity and Insulin Resistance

Having high insulin levels on a consistent basis means more body fat. Another important concept to be aware of is that not all body fat is the same, and when it comes to diabetes, of particular concern is a type of body fat often referred to as "visceral obesity."

Visceral obesity is a type of obesity in which fat is concentrated around the middle of the body, particularly surrounding the intestines. Visceral fat is linked to extra fat storage in the liver (which can raise blood sugar levels) and to extra fat in muscle cells, making them resistant to insulin.

Visceral obesity is evident when you have a waist measurement greater than the circumference of your hips. In most cases, individuals with visceral obesity have some degree of insulin resistance. One reason this happens is that extra adipose tissue ("fat") produces a hormone called resistin, which makes it harder for insulin to escort sugar into the cells.

In the following section, we will review how the cycle of insulin resistance builds and can lead to diabetes.

The Path to Insulin Resistance

Consistent consumption of sugar and fast-acting carbohydrates, combined with chronic high blood glucose levels and a large insulin response, sets the stage for an imbalanced state, as shown in the diagram below.

The Path to Insulin Resistance
Constantly eating foods that lead to rapid/large glucose & insulin spikes eventually can lead to a condition call insulin resistance which is a precursor to Type 2 Diabetes.

- It All Starts with Consuming Sugar & Fast Acting Carbs
  - Fast Sharp Rise of Blood Glucose
  - Large Insulin Response
  - Blood Glucose Levels Fall --- Often Sharply
  - Cravings Kick In
- Habits & Cravings Promote Consuming More Sugar & Fast Acting Carbs
  - Chronic Fast Sharp Rise of Blood Glucose Results in More Insulin Being Released
  - Cells Start to Become Insulin Resistant
  - Less Glucose is Moved Into Cells, Excess is Moved into Fat Storage as a Vicious Cycle of Cravings & Consuming Sugar Continues
- "Constant Hunger" May Be Experienced
- As cells become more insulin resistant, insulin moves less glucose into the cells
- **INSULIN RESISTANCE**
  - Pancreatic Alpha Cells React By Secreting More Glucagon & Blood Glucagon Levels Rise
  - The Liver & Muscles Breakdown Stored Glycogen to Release More Glucose Into the Blood
  - The Body Produces More Insulin to Try to Fix the Problem
  - Excess Fructose Adds to Insulin Resistance
  - Without Intervention, Insulin Resistance Worsens & Blood Glucose Levels Reamain High

- When your body is not responding fully to insulin, your cells absorb less glucose from your bloodstream, which causes you to have high blood glucose levels. This results in your cells utilizing less glucose.
- The pancreas reacts by producing more insulin. At the beginning of this cycle, the insulin response does several things. Insulin continues to try to transport and

store glucose into your cells. Insulin interacts with the surface of cells, but has difficulty opening the passageway, which subsequently prevents sufficient glucose from entering the cells, and insulin stores excess glucose in fat storage. The bottom line is that blood glucose levels fall.
- In response to falling glucose levels, your pancreatic alpha cells react by secreting more glucagon, and the glucagon levels in your blood rise.
- Glucagon then acts on your liver and muscles to break down stored glycogen and to release even more glucose into the blood, raising your blood glucose levels.
- Then this vicious cycle starts all over again. (The pancreas produces insulin, insulin-resistant cells take in a portion of the glucose, some glucose is stored as glycogen, and the excess is stored as fat. Glucose levels fall, glucagon prompts the breakdown of glycogen into glucose, which ends up in the bloodstream.)
- As the body tries to compensate, glucose and insulin levels swing from high to low and back again. Over the years, the weight gain increases, and the pancreas begins to exhaust itself.

As the situation worsens, your beta cells in the pancreas become "burned out" and are producing less insulin while struggling to keep up with ever-increasing blood glucose levels.

You might be wondering why the body's ability to store excess glucose in the muscles and liver as glycogen does not spare us from having high levels of glucose floating in our bloodstream. The problem is that the ability of our cells to store glycogen is not infinite. If glycogen starts to build up to high levels in the liver, the liver will repress additional synthesis. As a result, when more glucose continues to enter the liver cells, it is redirected into a different metabolic pathway.

With some simplification, here is what happens: Within this metabolic pathway, fatty acids are made and then transported out of the liver as ***lipoproteins***. While circulating, these lipoproteins are broken apart into free-floating fatty acids that are utilized by other tissues. Certain tissues in our body then use the fatty acids in order to make triglycerides.

The end result is that fats in the bloodstream are contributing to insulin resistance. Insulin resistance in turn causes elevated blood sugar and insulin levels, and elevated insulin levels cause the fat cells to build even more abdominal fat.

Ultimately, the imbalance leads to pre-diabetes or full-blown diabetes unless the process is interrupted by lifestyle changes or medication (or a combination of both) that can restore the body to a state of health.

Insulin Resistance and Hypoglycemia:

If you have insulin resistance and constantly eat foods like refined carbohydrates, a lot more insulin is needed to bring your blood sugar back down to healthy levels. Some people with insulin resistance produce so much insulin that their blood sugar levels dive way below normal, causing a condition called hypoglycemia. Hypoglycemia causes uncomfortable reactions such as jitteriness, tiredness, mental dullness, headaches, or intense cravings for sugary or starchy foods. Even though the hallmark of hypoglycemia is low blood sugar, and diabetes is characterized by high blood sugar, the root cause, i.e., the inability to process carbohydrates effectively, is the same. Many people who experience ongoing hypoglycemia later end up with Type 2 diabetes.

Why Weight Loss is Important

Experts note that even modest weight loss helps overcome insulin resistance and bring blood sugar levels down. In fact, many Type 2 diabetics find that the combination of losing weight and modest exercise enables them to reduce or eliminate their medications. Studies have shown that you can significantly lower your risk of getting full-blown diabetes by losing as little as 5-10% of your body weight and exercising as little as ½ hour per day.

Reaching and maintaining a reasonable weight is a component of your overall plan to improve your health, not because of societal pressure to look a certain way. But, if you have insulin resistance, prediabetes, or full-blown diabetes, weight loss helps you to control your blood glucose levels.

- When you lose weight, cells become more sensitive to insulin so that the body uses insulin more effectively.

- The result of more effective use of insulin is that insulin is able to move more glucose from the bloodstream into your cells.
- Your cells are now able to use the needed glucose for energy.
- The end result is an improvement in blood glucose levels, which for many diabetics means the ability to lower the dosage of glucose-lowering pills or, in some instances, eliminating medication or insulin injections.

If your weight is not within the guidelines for your height and age (check with your physician), consider weight loss as a key goal for your sugar-free lifestyle plan.

Pre-Diabetes and the Progression to Type 2 Diabetes

Insulin resistance is the foundation for the progression to pre-diabetes and type 2 diabetes.

Pre-diabetes is a condition characterized by blood sugar levels that are higher than normal but not yet high enough to be classified as type 2 diabetes. It typically begins with insulin resistance, where the body's cells become less responsive to insulin. This resistance leads to an increase in blood sugar levels, and over time, the pancreas may not be able to keep up with the increased demand for insulin, resulting in consistently elevated blood sugar levels. If left unmanaged, pre-diabetes can progress to type 2 diabetes.

Type 1 diabetes and type 2 diabetes have different causes, although both are characterized by elevated blood sugars and insulin problems.

Type 1 Diabetes: The pancreas either no longer produces insulin or doesn't produce enough of it.

Type 2 Diabetes: Your pancreas makes insulin, but you experience high glucose levels either because:

- The pancreas may not be producing insulin in sufficient quantity,
- The body's cells may have lost their ability to respond to insulin, even if the pancreas is producing enough insulin, or
- A combination of these two factors.

The Problem with Excess Glucose

When levels of glucose in the bloodstream get too high, blood cells can begin to cease to circulate as freely as they should. In effect, the blood of a diabetic becomes too "sticky." As a result, certain tissues can become seriously deprived of vital nutrients and oxygen. Damaging effects of excess glucose in the bloodstream include:

- **Cellular accumulation of sorbitol, a by-product of glucose metabolism.** High concentrations of glucose can lead to the cellular accumulation of sorbitol. The buildup of sorbitol within cells causes them to swell and damage tissue. This can lead to complications of the eyes and nerves.
- **Glycation.** This is a process by which glucose binds to, chemically alters, and damages proteins. This process results in the formation of advanced glycation end products referred to as "AGEs." AGEs form at a constant but slow rate in the normal body. Their formation, however, is markedly accelerated in uncontrolled diabetes because of the increased availability of glucose. Over time these altered proteins may accumulate in the cells and interfere with their normal functions. Complications of the eyes, kidneys, and circulatory system are associated with these altered proteins.
- **Increased production of free radicals.** Elevated levels of glucose increase the production of free radicals. Although free radicals are a natural by-product of normal cellular metabolism, free radical damage has been linked to heart disease, cancer, and other degenerative disorders.

Possible Diabetic Complications

The goal of any type of diabetes care is to keep blood sugar levels as normal as possible. As the following statistics from the American Diabetes Association show, uncontrolled diabetes can take an enormous toll .

- **Blindness.** The number one cause of blindness in people aged 2 to 70 is diabetic retinopathy. Glaucoma and cataracts are also more common in individuals with diabetes.

- **Kidney Failure**. Diabetes is the leading cause of kidney failure and is responsible for 40% of all new cases. .
- **Nerve Damage**. Diabetic neuropathy affects 60 to 70 percent of all diabetics. Symptoms range from mild loss of sensation in the feet to constant pain in various parts of the body. Nerve damage may also impair digestion and cause other complications.
- **Amputations**: Large numbers of amputations are performed every year on patients with diabetes, and it is a leading cause of non-traumatic amputations.
- **Cardiovascular disease**. Elevated blood sugar damages the blood vessels and alters blood lipid levels. High triglyceride levels are common in diabetics, as are low levels of protective HDL cholesterol. In addition, hypertension affects almost 60% of individuals with Type 2 diabetes. People who have diabetes are two to four times more likely to develop heart disease or have a stroke than non-diabetics, and three-fourths of all diabetics ultimately die of heart disease.

The treatment for Type 1 and Type 2 diabetes is also different, primarily because Type 1 is characterized by an inability of the pancreas to produce insulin. Treatment always includes replacing insulin via injections or pumps (in addition to patches and sprays currently being developed).

Treatment options for Type 2 diabetes may range from adjusting diet and exercise to taking oral medications, or in some cases, insulin is required. Early detection and lifestyle changes, such as improving diet, increasing physical activity, and losing weight, can help manage and potentially reverse pre-diabetes.

Even though treatment may differ, making lifestyle changes is critical for both Type 1 and Type 2 diabetes. It is true that Type 1 diabetics will always need to replace insulin, but with a good program of diet, exercise, and nutritional support, Type 1 diabetics will be able to more effectively manage their insulin use and avoid complications.

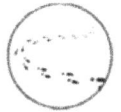

Action Steps

Learn How to Measure Your Waist to Recognize One of the First Signs of Insulin Resistance

Waist circumference is one of the most practical tools for assessing abdominal fat for signs of insulin resistance and chronic disease risk. For many people, one of the first signs of insulin resistance is excess weight around their middle, as insulin stores excess glucose as fat.

The fat surrounding the liver and other abdominal organs is very metabolically active. It releases fatty acids, inflammatory agents, and hormones, ultimately leading to higher LDL cholesterol, triglycerides, blood glucose, and blood pressure. A high waist circumference or a greater level of abdominal fat is associated with an increased risk for insulin resistance, type 2 diabetes, high cholesterol, high blood pressure, and heart disease.

Studies suggest that health risks begin to increase when a woman's waist reaches 31.5 inches, and her risk jumps substantially once her waist expands to 35 inches or more. For a man, risk starts to climb at 37 inches, but it becomes a bigger worry once his waist reaches or exceeds 40 inches. The waist circumference, where health becomes an issue, will vary based on your body type. The main thing is to be aware of changes in your body. For many people, an expanding waistline is one of the first signs of insulin resistance.

To properly measure your waist circumference:

- The tape measure should be placed directly on your skin or on no more than one layer of light clothing.
- The correct place to measure your waist is horizontally, halfway between your lowest rib and the top of your hipbone. This is roughly in line with your belly button

- Breathe out normally and take the measure. Make sure the tape is snug without squeezing the skin.

The most important next step to take is to discuss your findings with your physician so that, together, you can plan a course of action to further assess your health and take steps to reverse insulin resistance and reduce your risk for chronic illness.

Speak with Your Physician if You Have Symptoms of Insulin Resistance

Below is a list of some of the most common symptoms of insulin resistance, a precursor to diabetes. It is very possible to affect the progression of diabetes by making lifestyle changes. If you are experiencing one or more of these symptoms, speak with your physician, especially if you have risk factors for diabetes.

- **Fatigue**. The failure of insulin to work properly and the inability of your cells to get sufficient glucose eventually take their toll on the body. Some people with insulin resistance are tired in the morning or afternoon. Others are exhausted all day.
- **Low blood sugar**. Prolonged periods of hypoglycemia, accompanied by many of the symptoms listed here, especially physical and mental fatigue, may be symptoms of insulin resistance.
- **Sleepiness**. Many people with insulin resistance get sleepy immediately after eating a meal containing more than 20% or 30% carbohydrates. This is often a pasta meal, or even a meat meal that includes potatoes or bread, and a sweet dessert.
- **Increased weight and fat storage**. In males, a large abdomen is the more obvious and earliest sign of insulin resistance. In females, it can be a large abdomen and/or prominent buttocks.
- **Increased triglycerides**. Individuals typically may have stores of excess triglycerides in their arteries as a result of insulin resistance.

Know the Risk Factors for Diabetes

If you have any of the following risk factors, you may be at an increased risk for diabetes. You should be particularly vigilant about the symptoms of diabetes and discuss any concerns you have with your physician.

- Family History
- Diabetes during pregnancy or had a baby
- 20% over a healthy weight or obese
- weighing 9 lb. or more at birth
- Sedentary Lifestyle
- Low HDL (good cholesterol) or high overall cholesterol levels
- You are African American, Latino, Asian, Native American or Pacific Islander
- Very high blood pressure or very high triglycerides

Discuss Testing with Your Physician if You are Experiencing Symptoms of Diabetes

Diabetes has several symptoms that you might not suspect are associated with the disease. If you experience one or more of the symptoms below, discuss diabetes testing with your healthcare provider.

- Frequent urination
- Excessive thirst
- Unexplained weight loss
- Unusual hunger
- Extreme fatigue
- Irritability
- Frequent infections
- Blurred vision
- Slow to heal cuts and bruises
- Vaginitis or recurring yeast infections in women
- Tingling or numbness in hands or feet
- Recurring skin, gum or bladder infections

Takeaways & Highlights

Learning how your body works gives you the knowledge to make decisions that empower you to eat in a way that:

- Works in harmony with your unique biochemistry,
- Keeps your blood sugar and insulin levels in a balanced state,
- Eliminates your personal trigger foods,
- Conquers cravings, and
- Helps you to stick with it for the long term.

Our cells need energy in the form of glucose, and your body gets the glucose it requires from the food you eat, primarily from carbohydrates.

Glucose has to be delivered to and absorbed by your cells for it to do any good, and there is a delicate balance of insulin and blood sugar that needs to be maintained in order for your body to function properly.

Carbohydrates are not foods but rather collections of molecules consisting of carbon, oxygen, and hydrogen. Chemically, at their most basic level, ALL carbohydrates are made up of units of sugar. These sugar units are called saccharide units.

- There are two main classifications of carbohydrates: Simple sugars and complex carbohydrates. Starches and cellulose are two types of complex carbohydrates.
- The digestive system processes carbohydrates, breaking them down into glucose, so that the carbohydrates are converted into a form that is usable by our cells.
- Insulin transports glucose in the blood to cells in our muscles and other parts of the body for use in energy production or storage as fat.

When the body's digestive and related self-regulating mechanisms break down anywhere in the process, over time, insulin resistance, diabetes, and other chronic conditions result. Risk factors for type 2 diabetes include:

- Family history
- 20% over a healthy weight or obese
- Sedentary Lifestyle
- You are African American, Latino, Asian, Native American, or Pacific Islander
- Diabetes during pregnancy or you gave birth to a baby weighing 9 pounds or more
- Low HDL (good cholesterol) or high overall cholesterol levels
- Very high blood pressure or triglyceride levels

Lifestyle changes, including maintaining a sugar-free lifestyle, can be a powerful way to conquer insulin resistance, pre-diabetes, and/or diabetes. Type 1 diabetes always requires the administration of insulin, but lifestyle changes can greatly impact the amount of insulin needed and overall health.

CHAPTER 12
Implement a Food Plan that Eliminates Personal Trigger Foods

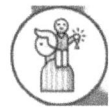

Coach on Your Shoulder

Maintaining a Sugar-Free Lifestyle is Not the Same Thing as Going on a Diet

The Sugar-Free Lifestyle Food Plan is designed to help you develop a personalized food plan that reflects your self-motivated vision of how you want to eat to support your health. Using this plan, you can determine what you want to eat, when you want to eat, and how much of certain foods you want to consume on a day-to-day basis. It is a guide for eating and living in harmony with your body functions, and creating a personalized food plan that works for your unique biochemistry.

The Benefits of Using a Food Plan to Eat in Harmony with How Your Body Works

In this chapter, you are going to learn how to change your body composition through a plan based on how your body works. The goal is to empower you to create a sugar-free lifestyle with a balanced physical state that allows your body's mechanisms to function in harmony without following strict menus or counting, weighing, and measuring.

Many programs can be challenging to follow, and after a while, most dieters tend to give up. The Sugar-Free Lifestyle Food Plan™ is based on several straightforward concepts designed to help you stick with and get results, including:

- Eat more non-starchy vegetables and protein,
- Include healthy fats, and
- Eliminate added sugar and trigger foods that cause sharp/ fast increases in glucose and insulin levels.

This plan enables you to select foods from a wide variety of sources based on your unique biochemistry and food preferences.

Learning to eat in harmony with how your body works has many benefits, including:

- You are eating foods that do not result in a fast/sharp rise in blood glucose levels
- Your body's insulin response is moderated
- You gain control of your blood sugar levels and eliminate any insulin resistance
- You are able to conquer physical cravings for sugar from various sources (added, natural, and hidden)
- You can eliminate personal trigger foods and stay on track for the long term

Why a Food Plan is different than a "diet"

There are many reasons that dieting does not work for the majority of people, which explains why so many Americans experience yo-yo dieting and frustration. Traditional diet approaches do not attack the underlying causes of sugar addiction or blood sugar health issues. Instead, they tell you to have willpower, to count calories or carbs, to eat very restrictively, and to exercise more. As a result, most people achieve temporary results. Sooner or later, cravings and roller-coaster blood sugar levels return because the roadblocks preventing individuals from successfully maintaining a sugar-free lifestyle were never eliminated.

Below are some of the key reasons why going on a diet is not a helpful option to conquer sugar and related blood sugar health issues, including insulin resistance, pre-diabetes, and full-blown diabetes.

- **Diets are temporary**. Most diets do not teach you how to eat for life. Instead, they offer you a quick fix that is not attainable over the long term.
- **Diets distort your relationship with food**. Very importantly, diets teach you not to listen to your body. Instead, they instruct you to follow rigid menus, count calories, measure your food, and in general, to ignore your hunger with will power.
- **Diets lead to boredom and frustration**. People often get bored or frustrated with diets and begin to cheat "just a little," and then soon abandon the diet.
- **When you diet, you are likely to lose muscle and gain body fat**. When you go back to your old habits, you will gain back the muscle you've lost as body fat, and this, in turn, contributes to the vicious cycle of insulin resistance.

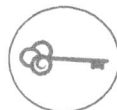

Key Concepts

Adopting a Quality Carbohydrate Approach vs. Low Carb or Keto

Of all the foods in your plan, the amount and type of carbohydrates that you eat will have the most dramatic impact on your blood sugar levels. Understanding how carbohydrates function in your body will help you make informed choices that support normal blood sugar levels.

- Keep in mind that you are not going to avoid all carbohydrates. To the contrary, if you keep the following guiding principle in mind when selecting carbohydrates, you will rarely go wrong: "the longer your body has to wrestle with a carbohydrate to break it down into glucose, the slower the rise in glucose in your blood."
- The key to including carbohydrates in your diet is remembering that not all carbohydrates are created equal.

- You want to strive to include good quality complex carbohydrates in your food plan that are 1) unrefined, 2) nutritious, 3) high in fiber, and 4) do not contribute to dramatic swings in your blood sugar and subsequent spiked insulin responses.

Choosing to eat (or reject) a food based on the amount of carbohydrate it contains only gives you a small piece of the carbohydrate puzzle. In order to successfully manage blood sugars, a number of factors should be considered, including the type of carbohydrate, the amount of processing, and the amount of carbohydrate consumed.

The Sugar-Free Lifestyle Food Plan™ is a Quality Carbohydrate plan that focuses on eliminating carbohydrates that cause fast/sharp rises in blood glucose levels while including carbohydrates that provide needed nutrition and moderate blood sugar and insulin levels. The plan does not rely on carb counting but does incorporate some aspects of low-carb food plans, which actually exist on a continuum from very low (Keto) to more moderate amounts of carbohydrates.

There is no definitive definition for what constitutes low-carb. What is low-carbohydrate for one person may not be for another.

Basically, all low-carb food plans are designed to reduce the number of carbs you eat from your normal diet. As a general rule, however, a low-carb diet typically includes anywhere from 50 to 100 grams (g) of carbohydrates per day. Below that amount is considered a ketogenic diet, while 100 to 200 grams of carbohydrates per day is generally considered a moderate-carb diet.

Some plans are based on "net carbs" (total carbohydrate amount minus fiber + sugar alcohols*), while others calculate daily carbohydrates based on the total carbohydrate amount.

*NOTE: Some plans only permit subtracting the full amount of the sugar alcohol erythritol (and ½ of any other sugar alcohol such as maltitol).

The Sugar-Free Lifestyle Food Plan™ is not designed to put you in a state of Ketosis. It is recommended that if you desire to consume the grams of carbs

required for you to be in a state of Ketosis, you work with your physician to do so.

Tips for Making the Food Plan Work for You

- **Keep it simple**. Any plan that is overly complicated will soon be discarded, and before you know it, you will be back to your old eating habits. If you develop an easy-to-implement food plan, you will find that making food choices within the context of the plan will become second nature.
- **Balance consistency with flexibility**. Planning what you will eat daily will enable you to avoid the pitfalls of impulse eating. The more predictable your food intake is, the more predictable your glucose levels are going to be, and you are less likely to experience cravings and chaotic food choices.
- **Develop a plan that fits your lifestyle and aligns with your overall vision of health**. It is critical that your food plan fits your lifestyle and particular needs. For example, if you are a vegetarian, you will want to incorporate ways to obtain protein from sources other than animal foods. If you have a hectic professional life or frequently eat on the go, you need to consider these situations.
- **If you are diabetic, check your blood sugar levels**. The bottom line is that it doesn't matter whether you are told you can or cannot eat a particular food. All that matters is how your body reacts to it. If you experience a rapid rise in blood sugar levels soon after a food is consumed or your blood sugars remain high 1-2 hours after eating, it is not a good choice for you. Even if you are not diabetic, your body will give you clues if you have experienced a blood sugar spike followed by a crash. Did you feel tired or sleepy after eating, or did you find yourself experiencing cravings the rest of the day?

The Sugar-Free Lifestyle Food Plan™ Success Strategies

As you create your daily food plan, remember that a particular food is not inherently good or bad, and there is no perfect way to maintain a sugar-free lifestyle. Based on your unique goals, physical condition, and biochemistry, you can select or leave out any of the foods in the recommended list of options. You should avoid personal trigger foods or foods that cause a fast and sharp rise in blood sugar levels.

The reality is that there is no perfect way to eat. Everyone metabolizes food slightly differently. You will know what works for you based on your own results (i.e. blood sugar levels based on daily monitoring, weight loss, your energy levels, etc.).

That being said, there are some guiding principles that will help you to manage your blood sugar levels as well as cholesterol and triglyceride levels. Your food plan should also help you to maintain a desirable weight, consume adequate nutrients, and diminish cravings.

The Food Plan provides strategies for optimizing your food plan. They are meant to be flexible, and it is important to avoid a rigid attitude towards food that can hinder your ability to stick with it. With the following guidelines in mind, you can develop a personalized daily food plan that meets your individual needs.

Crowd Out Foods that Cause a Fast/Sharp Rise in Blood Glucose Levels

- Eliminate added sugar. Stop adding sugar to beverages and recipes, and replace processed foods containing added sugar with no-sugar-added alternatives.
- Eliminate hidden sugar, which are foods that behave like simple sugars during the digestion process and cause a sharp/fast rise in blood glucose levels. These foods include:
    - Grain-Based Flour Products
    - White Potatoes
    - Rice
- Cut back on fruit and the natural sugar fructose.
- Go easy on the natural sugar lactose.

Eliminate Personal Trigger Foods

- Identify your personal trigger foods
- Eliminate personal trigger foods from your kitchen and food plan

Nourish Your Body with Foods that Support Vibrant Health

- Change your plate and develop a daily food plan that is based on:
    - 50% non-starchy vegetables
    - 25% healthy protein
    - 25% combo of healthy fats and quality carbohydrates
    - Increased fiber. Try to include at least 25-30 grams of fiber daily.

Stay Hydrated

- Consume enough water and other healthy liquids

Adopt New Habits That Improve HOW You Eat

- Watch portion sizes.
- Eat mindfully.
- Be aware of your eating schedule and avoid nighttime eating.
- Snack smart.
- Build a better breakfast.
- Make food prep easier.

Food Plan Overview and Sugar-Free Lifestyle Food List

This section provides an overview of food choices for daily meals and snack planning, based on the Food Plan guidelines and Action Steps.

Now that you know what happens inside your body when you consistently eat foods that cause fast/sharp rises in blood glucose levels, it will come as no surprise that creating a food plan that avoids carbohydrates and sugar sources that can quickly raise blood glucose levels is a core principle for maintaining a sugar-free lifestyle.

Food Plan Overview

Eliminate "Added Sugar"

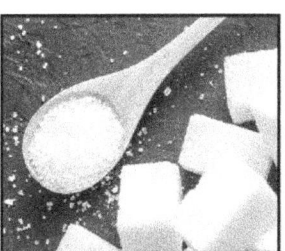

Eliminate/Avoid Grain-Based Flour Products

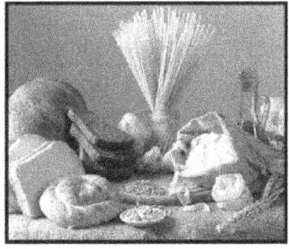

Based on your biochemistry & trigger foods you can include small amounts of:

- Starchy Vegetables (squash, sweet potatoes, peas, etc.)

- Dairy (low in lactose)

- Dark Chocolate (no sugar)

- Sweeteners of Choice, such as Stevia, Monkfruit. & Allulose

Eliminate/Avoid White Potatoes

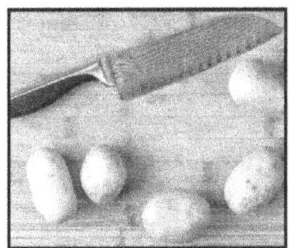

Eliminate/Avoid Rice

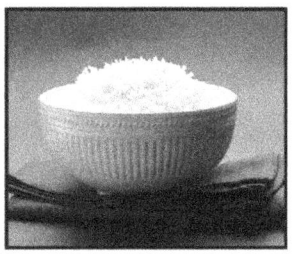

Go Easy on Foods with "Natural Sugars"

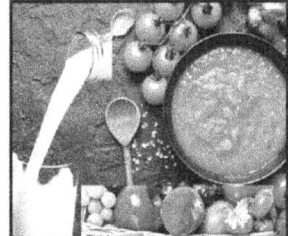

Choose Low Glycemic Fruit

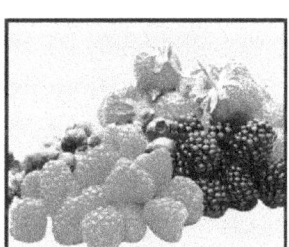

Drink Water & Other Blood Sugar Friendly Beverages

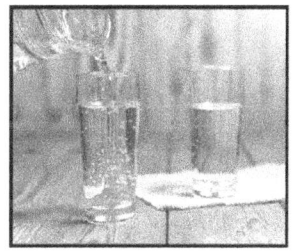

Focus on Non-Starchy Vegetables, Healthy Protein & Healthy Fats

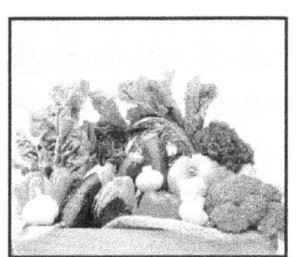
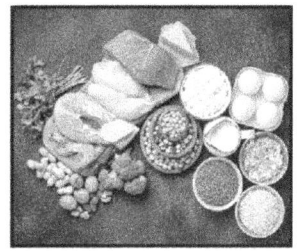
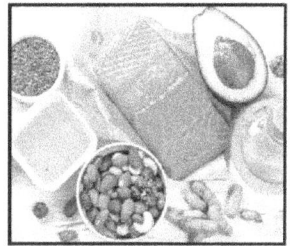

Food Plan List

Non-Starchy Vegetables		
Green: Alfalfa sprouts, Artichokes, Arugula, Asparagus, Broccoli, Broccolini, Bok Choy, Broccoli Rabe, Brussels Sprouts, Celery, Cucumbers, Endive, Fennel, Green Beans, Green Bell Peppers, Green Cabbage, Leeks, Okra, Snow Peas, Scallions, Spinach, Watercress, Zucchini **Leafy Greens/Lettuce** (Arugula, Bib Lettuce, Butterhead Lettuce, Collard Greens, Dandelion Greens, Endive, Iceberg Lettuce, Kale, Mesclun, Romaine Lettuce, Parsley, Swiss Chard, Watercress)	**Red:** Radicchio, Radishes, Red Okra, Red Onions, Red Peppers, Rhubarb, Tomatoes (whole and small cherry tomatoes) **Orange:** Carrots, Rutabagas, Yellow & Orange Bell Peppers, Yellow Summer Squash **Purple:** Eggplant, Purple Cabbage **White:** Cauliflower, Garlic, Ginger, Hearts of Palm, Jerusalem Artichokes, Jicama, Kohlrabi, Mushrooms, Onions, Sauerkraut, Shallots, Water Chestnuts	**Marine Plants:** (Arame, Dulse, Hijiki, Irish Moss, Kelp, Kombu, Nori, Sea Lettuce, Wakame) **Technically Fruits:** (Avocado, Hot Peppers, Olives)
Healthy Protein		
Beef: (Lean, Grass Fed) **Fish:** (Best: High Eco Rating, low mercury content, high Omega 3 content) Examples: Wild Salmon, Sardines, Herring, Sablefish, Albacore Tuna from U.S./Canada **Pork:** (Lean) (Occasional Bacon) **Poultry:** (Organic, Free Range) **Shellfish & Other Seafood:** (Calamari, Lobster, Oysters, Mussels, Shrimp)	**Legumes:** (Canned or Dried – Includes Lentils and Beans) **Beans:** (Adzuki, Anasazi, Black, Black-eyed peas, Borlotti, Cannellini, Chickpea, Edamame, Fava, Flageolet, Great Northern, Lima, Lupin, Kidney, Mung, Navy, Pink, Pinto, Soybeans) **Lentils:** (Brown, Green, Red/Yellow, French, Black Beluga)	**Eggs:** (Best: Pasture Raised) Protein Powder: (Casein, Collagen, Egg White, Hemp, Pea, Rice, Soy, Whey Isolate or Isolate/Concentrate) **Tempeh** **Tofu**

Dairy (source of protein, carbohydrates, and fats) Best: No Added Sugar, Low Lactose, Fat % choice determined by your biochemistry and state of health		
Butter: (Grass Fed) **Coconut Creme** **Cream Cheese** **Cottage Cheese** **Ghee** **Mascarpone** **Ricotta Cheese** **Sour Cream** **Yogur**t (No Added Sugar Greek, Skyre--- Source: Cow's Milk, Goat's Milk, or Plant/Nut Alternative)	<u>**Cow's Milk or No Added Sugar Plant/Nut Alternatives**</u>: (Almond, Oat, Cashew, Coconut, Hazelnut, Hemp, Macadamia, Soy, Walnut) **Goat's Milk** **Kefir:** (No Added Sugar- Cow's Milk, Goat's Milk, or Plant/Nut Alternative)	<u>**Hard/Soft Cheeses**</u>: (Blue, Brie, Colby, Cheddar, Feta, Goat, Gorgonzola, Gouda, Mozzarella, Muenster, Parmesan, Provolone, Swiss)
Healthy Fats		
<u>**Oils:**</u> (Avocado, Coconut, Olive, or oils from Nuts/Seeds Listed in the Food Plan List)	<u>**Nuts:**</u> (Almonds, Brazil, Hazelnuts, Macadamia, Peanuts, Pecans, Pine Nuts, Pistachios, Walnuts) <u>**Occasiona**</u>l: Cashews	<u>**Seeds:**</u> (Chia, Flax, Hemp, Psyllium, Poppy, Pumpkin, Sunflower, Sesame, Poppy) **Nut/Seed Butter:** (No Sugar Added from nuts & seeds listed in the Food Plan List)
Starchy Vegetables, Grains, Chocolate & Sweeteners		
<u>**Winter Squash**</u>: (Acorn, Buttercup, Butternut, Delicata, Hubbard, Kabocha, Pumpkin, Red Kuri, Spaghetti)	<u>**Quinoa:**</u> (technically a seed, but often used as a substitute for rice) **Occasional:** Barley, Buckwheat, Steel Cut Oats, Sprouted Grain Bread	<u>**Chocolate**</u>: Minimum 60% Cacao, no sugar added (small amount occasionally) <u>**Sugar Alternatives**</u>: (Monk Fruit, Stevia, or another sugar-free source based on preference)
Fruit		
<u>**Low Glycemic Berries**</u>: (Berries Strawberries, Blueberries, Raspberries, Blackberries)	<u>**Other Low Glycemic Fruit**</u>: (Avocado, Coconut, Lemons, Limes)	<u>**Occasional Choices**</u>: (See Fruit Chart in Appendix)

Putting it All Together: Meal Planning

Ideally, 75% of your daily food intake should consist of non-starchy vegetables and high-quality protein. But, for long-term success, remember that eating is not a science.

50%	25%	25%	Occasional
Non starchy VEGETABLES (raw or cooked) +	High Quality Protein (You can consume less protein, add some extra non-starchy vegetables) +	Starchy Vegetables Low GI Fruits Healthy Fats Nuts/Seeds	Dairy Cheese Alternative Sweeteners Non-grain based flour Chocolate Medium GI fruit

Each day, strive to stay as close to the Sugar-Free Lifestyle Food Plan™ as possible. However, you don't have to be exact, and you don't have to give up enjoying all your favorite foods or follow a plan of deprivation.

One food category that is highly personal to most people is the type and amount of protein they consume. You can customize your protein based on your eating style, including whether you are carnivorous, pescatarian, vegetarian, vegan, or a combination of any of these. You can also adjust the amount of protein and modify your vegetable consumption accordingly.

Another way to approach menu planning is to visualize what your plate might look like at each meal, based on the percentages shown in the diagram above. It is deliberately a simple plan. There is no need to count or measure. Just keep an eye on the percentages, watch portion sizes, and be extra vigilant with personal trigger foods. If you are planning a one-pot meal, such as a stew or a dish with multiple ingredients, such as a stir fry, estimate the percentages of the ingredients and add a salad for good measure.

*NOTE: Breakfast is one meal where you might not consume as many vegetables, but try to include a serving of vegetables at least 3-5 times per week.

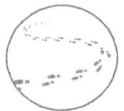

Action Steps

Eliminate Added Sugar

Added sugar includes sugar added to foods during preparation and processing. The Food Plan Daily Food List does not include any foods with added sugar. When you select foods from this list, read labels to avoid brands of processed foods with added sugar and refrain from using added sugar in food preparation. Whether you choose to occasionally consume foods that contain 1 gram or less of added sugar depends on your health goals, unique biochemistry, and trigger foods. If you have diabetes, pre-diabetes, or insulin resistance, it is strongly recommended that you eliminate all added sugar. Likewise, if you have a physical or emotional addiction to sugar, added sugar is best avoided, including any trigger foods containing added sugar.

We covered the topic of Eliminating Added Sugar in Phase 1. If you have not completed the Action Steps found in Chapter 9 or want to revisit them, the Action Steps include:

- Read Labels to Find Added Sugar
- Stop Adding Sugar to food, recipes, and beverages
- Learn About Alternative Sweeteners
- Eliminate Soda (including diet)
- Replace Salad Dressings that Contain Added Sugar
- Replace Yogurt Containing Added Sugar with Plain Yogurt (and Flavor the Yogurt Yourself
- Replace High Sugar Smoothies with No Added Sugar/Low Natural Sugar Alternatives
- Replace pantry items (such as condiments, canned goods, sauces, etc.) with brands that contain no added sugar.

Eliminate Hidden Sugar Sources

Not all complex carbohydrates behave the way you expect them to. For example, grain-based flour products, rice, and starchy vegetables, like white potatoes, behave more like simple sugars during the digestion process, breaking down quickly into glucose and causing a sharp rise in blood glucose levels along with a large insulin response. I refer to these foods as "hidden sugar." Sources. To maximize your efforts, avoid hidden sugars and choose complex carbohydrates that release glucose more slowly into the bloodstream

Cutting Back on Whole Grains, Rice, and Potatoes

Not all complex carbohydrates behave the way you expect them to. Consume certain whole grains very judiciously and avoid starchy vegetables such as white potatoes. White potatoes and certain grains behave more like simple sugars, breaking down quickly into glucose and causing a sharp insulin response.

If you choose to include grains in your food plan, the best choices are cooked whole grains such as quinoa, oats, barley, or rye. Quinoa is often considered to be a grain, but it is actually a seed.

White rice should be avoided, and brown rice can be consumed occasionally, in very small quantities, unless it is a trigger food or if it causes a fast, sharp rise in your blood sugar levels.

The Problem With Grain-based Flour Products

It is best to avoid all grain-based flour products as well as gluten-free flour made with potato or rice flour.

- Grinding grains into flour increases the surface area upon which enzymes work to more quickly convert starch into glucose. This means that any grain-based flour products have the same effect on blood sugar, whether the flour is produced from whole grains or not.
- Sprouted grain products are digested more like a vegetable with slower digestion and less of a spike in blood sugar. Sprouted grain breads will not have "flour" in the ingredients, but should still be eaten in moderation.

- If you are diabetic, you should check your blood sugar levels after eating grains or grain-based products to confirm their effect on your blood sugar levels.
- Best breads: Non-grain based flour breads (made with nut, bean, golden flax meal, or coconut flour and occasional sprouted whole grain breads

When reading labels of bread products, look for the word flour in the ingredients. If a food product contains flour from a grain, avoid it. This includes any product traditionally containing grain-based flour, such as bread, muffins, tortillas, wraps, pancakes, waffles, crackers, cakes, and snack chips. This does not mean that you can never eat bread, crackers, or breakfast foods such as pancakes or waffles. Below are some alternatives. The only foods that should be avoided entirely, even in an alternative form, are trigger foods.

Bread, Wraps, Tortillas, Flatbreads, English Muffins, and Pasta Options:

- Purchase products made with an alternative flour (nut flour, bean flour, coconut flour, ground flax meal).
- Use Sprouted Grain Products that do not have flour in the ingredients. (Sprouted grain products are digested more like a vegetable with less of a spike in blood sugar levels).
- Try an alternative to bread, such as lettuce wraps, in place of bread for sandwiches.
- Explore pasta alternatives made with alternatives to grain-based flour, including "noodles" made with egg whites and egg white wraps that can be used in place of lasagna noodles. (Two popular brands are "Egglife" and "Crepini")

Crackers and Chips Options:

- Make your own from no-grain-based flour flatbreads, wraps, or tortillas.
- Buy store-bought brands that contain no grain-based flour.
- Use vegetables instead of crackers or chips (cucumber or zucchini rounds, carrot chips, red/yellow/green pepper slices, cherry tomatoes, broccoli or cauliflower florets).

Pancakes and Waffle Options:

- Make your own pancakes and waffles with a no-grain-based flour recipe or a store-bought product that contains no grain-based flour.
- Make chaffles with ingredients that typically include eggs, cheese, and flavorings of choice (some recipes also include a small amount of no-grain-based flour).

Cut Back on Fruit and the Natural Sugar Fructose

Most fruits contain a combination of several natural sugars, including glucose, sucrose, and fructose. For example, one cup of raw blueberries (approximately 148 grams) contains the following types and amounts of sugar:

- Total Sugars: 14.74 grams
- Fructose: 6.76 grams
- Glucose: 6.06 grams
- Sucrose: 1.36 grams

These figures are approximate, as the precise amounts of each sugar can vary depending on factors such as the specific variety of blueberry, growing conditions, and degree of ripeness (Source: USDA's National Nutrient Database).

Unlike glucose, fructose is primarily metabolized in the liver, and its processing does not raise blood sugar levels in the same way as glucose or stimulate insulin secretion significantly. This is why whole fruits that contain fiber and other healthy nutrients are included in many diet programs. Although fructose can be converted into glucose or glycogen, it also triggers something called "lipogenesis" (the process of converting excess carbohydrates into fatty acids in the liver and adipose tissue).

These fatty acids can then be converted into triglycerides for storage, and excessive consumption of fructose can have a propensity to increase triglyceride levels. New studies also show a link between high fructose consumption and insulin resistance.

When it comes to fruit, moderation is the best approach. You don't have to avoid all fruit, but be aware of both the amount and type of sugar as you make decisions about which fruits and the amount to include in your food plan. If you are insulin resistant, diabetic, have high cholesterol, and/or high triglycerides, it is best to limit your intake of fruit and fructose. I often tell my clients to include fruit like you would a condiment, for example, as a topping or added to a salad for a touch of sweetness. As fruit ripens, the overall amount of carbohydrates does not change. However, the sugar content increases as more starches turn to sugar. So, while ripe fruits taste delicious, be aware that they will have a higher sugar content. Below are recommended fruits to enjoy and those to avoid, followed by a chart to help you select fruit for consumption.

BEST choices for normalizing blood sugars and crushing cravings:

- Lemons, limes
- Avocados
- Berries (Strawberries, Blueberries, Raspberries, Blackberries)
- Unsweetened acai (frozen or powder)

BETTER options than high glycemic fruit choices (in moderation):

- Non-ripe banana (1/2-1/4)
- Apples, pears (slice and try to eat with some protein)
- Oranges, grapefruits
- Grapes, cherries, kiwi, mango, peaches
- Watermelon

AVOID:

- Ripe bananas
- Pineapple
- Dried fruit, raisins
- Very ripe cantaloupe, honey dew

Fruit Consumption Guide

Source: Nutrition Data: Know What You Eat [USDA SR-21

Fruit/Amount	Carbs (grams)	Fiber (Grams)	Starches (grams)	Sugars (grams)	Sucrose	Glucose	Fructose	Glycemic Load
BEST								
Avocado 1 cup cubed (150 grams)	12.8	10.1	0.2	1 g	90 mg	555 mg	180 mg	3
Avocado 1 cup pureed (230 grams)	19.6	15.4	0.3	1.5	138 mg	851 mg	276 mg	4
Lemon 1 Medium (58 Grams)	5.4	1.6	0.0	1.5	No Data	No Data	No Data	1
Lime 1 Small/Medium								
Tomato 1 Medium (123 grams)	4.8	1.5	0.0	3.2	0.0	1537 mg	1685 mg	2
Strawberries ½-3/4 cup Raw (100 grams)	7.7	2 g	0.0	4.9	470 g	1990 mg	2440 mg	2
Blackberries ½-3/4 cup (100 Grams)	10.2	5.3	0.0	4.9	70 mg	2310 mg	2400 mg	3
Blueberries 50 Berries raw (68 Grams)	9.9	1.6	0.0	6.8	74.8 mg	3318 mg	3379 mg	3
Raspberries 1 cup whole raw (123 grams)	14.7	8 g	0.0	5.4	246 mg	2288 mg	2890 mg	3
CONSUME OCCASIONALLY								
Grapefruit ½ raw (small -123 grams)	13.1	2	0.0	8.5	4317 mg	1980 mg	2177 mg	4
Orange 1 small 2-3/8 in diam (96 grams)	11.3	2.3	0.0	9.0	No Data	No Data	No Data	3

Fruit/Amount	Carbs (grams)	Fiber (Grams)	Starches (grams)	Sugars (grams)	Sucrose	Glucose	Fructose	Glycemic Load
Watermelon 1 cup diced (152 grams)	11.5	0.6	0.0	9.4	1839 mg	2402 mg	5106 mg	3
Peach 1 small (2 ½ in dia-130 grams)	12.9	1.9	0.0	10.9	6189 mg	2535 mg	1989 mg	4
Apple 1 cup slices (109 grams)	15.1	2.6	0.1	11.3	2257 mg	2649 mg	6431 mg	3
AVOID OR CONSUME SPARINGLY								
Banana (small) 101 grams	23.1	2.6	5.4	12.4	2414 mg	5029 mg	4898 mg	8
Cantaloupe 1 Cup Cubes (160 grams)	14.1	1.4	0.0	12.6	6959 mg	2464 mg	2992 mg	4
Honeydew 1 Cup Cubes (170 Grams)	15.5	1.4	0.0	13.8	4216 mg	4557 mg	5032mg	4
Pear Raw 1 small (148 Grams)	22.9	4.6	0.0	14.5	1154 mg	4085 m	9222 mg	5
Pineapple 1 cup chunks (165 grams)	21.6	2.3	0.0	16.3	9883 mg	2855 mg	3498mg	6
Watermelon 1 Wedge (approx. 1/16 of melon) (286 Grams)	21.6	1.1	0.0	17.7	3461 mg	4519m g	9608 mg	6
Cherries 1 cup with pits (138 grams)	22.1	2.9	0.0	17.7	207 mg	9093 mg	7410 mg	7
Grapes 1 cup Thompson Seedless (151 Grams)	27.3	1.4	0.0	23.4	227 mg	10872mg	12276 mg	9
Mango 1 cup sliced (165 grams)	28.1	3	0.0	24.4	No Data	No Data	No Data	8

Go Easy on Dairy Foods that Contain the Natural Sugar Lactose

Dairy Foods Overview

There are several types of dairy products, including:

- Milk: the base form of dairy products (Whole, 2%, 1%, Skim).
- Cream: the high-fat layer skimmed from the top of milk.
- Butter: made by separating butterfat from the buttermilk in cream.
- Cheese: made by coagulating one of the proteins in milk called casein.
- Yogurt: made by fermenting either milk or cream to convert milk sugar into lactic acid.
- Kefir: Kefir is a fermented dairy product that is made by mixing 'kefir grains,' composed of a complex structure of bacteria and yeasts with proteins, lipids, and sugars, with milk. The microorganisms ferment the naturally occurring milk sugar, lactose, into a sour, carbonated beverage with a consistency similar to thin yogurt.

Dairy foods are a source of:

- **Carbohydrate**. This includes natural sugar lactose.
- **Fat**. The amount of fat varies and affects the way dairy foods/lactose are metabolized.
- **Protein**. Dairy protein includes casein, which is digested slowly and provides a steady release of amino acids into the bloodstream, and whey, which is digested faster than casein.

How Lactose Affects Cravings and Blood Sugar Levels

Chemically, lactose is a disaccharide composed of two simpler sugars: glucose and galactose. It's primarily responsible for the subtle sweetness inherent in fresh milk. Lactose molecules break down when they arrive in the small intestine as part of the digestion process. An enzyme called lactase splits lactose into the smaller molecules: glucose and galactose. For many people, lactose is easily digestible; however, a significant portion of the global population lacks sufficient levels of the enzyme lactase, and as a result, they can experience lactose intolerance, leading to various digestive discomforts.

Many people can tolerate small amounts of the natural sugar lactose in their food plan without negative effects, while for others, even a small amount will trigger cravings and blood sugar spikes. Three factors determine the impact of lactose on your glucose and insulin levels immediately and over time.

- The amount of protein and fat contained in the dairy product or other foods that are eaten along with the dairy product. (Fat and protein typically help glucose enter the bloodstream more slowly and steadily, blunting fast/sharp blood sugar and insulin spikes).
- The amount of lactose in the dairy product (and the amount of any added or hidden sugars)
- Your biochemistry and unique response to sugar/lactose

Knowing your health goals and having clarity about your trigger foods will help you determine whether to consume lactose and the amount to include in your food plan. The bottom line is that it's best to consume dairy and lactose in moderation. If you have health concerns or are being treated for diabetes or any type of heart disease, talk to your physician about the best approach to consuming dairy for your particular health issues.

Eliminate Personal Trigger Foods, and Complete the Trigger Foods Worksheet

As we discussed in earlier chapters, the drive to food is both physical and psychological. Physically, sugar can lead to the release of dopamine in our brain, triggering feelings of pleasure, which makes it addictive. Additionally, eating a diet of foods that cause fast/sharp spikes in glucose and insulin can result in both roller coaster blood sugar levels and insulin resistance.

The desire for trigger foods is a complex process that progresses over time and, for many individuals, reaches a point where a pattern emerges of eating trigger foods that drive physical cravings for either more of the same food or that lead to cravings and binging on other foods. This starts a continuing cascade of high blood sugar levels along with the release of dopamine, sharp/fast releases of insulin, followed by crashes that leave individuals hungry for more sugar, not to mention the desire for another dopamine hit.

Many times, people do not even realize that they are eating trigger foods and can't understand why their cravings do not go away or get worse. The bottom line is that unless your personal trigger foods are eliminated, no amount of willpower will stop the cycle. You might be able to suck it up and use willpower to follow a diet for a week or even months. But if food triggers are introduced knowingly or unknowingly, the cravings will reappear.

If you want to quit sugar for the long term and get roller coaster blood sugars and cravings under control, it is critical to eliminate personal trigger foods. For most people, that means all added sugars, and then figuring out what other foods are trigger foods for you.

We all have a unique biochemistry, and so you can't rely on an expert's blanket statement that fruit, sugar substitutes, bread, grains, or any other food is OK or, alternatively, must be avoided. The real question is, how does that food affect you? It may take a little detective work, but identifying and eliminating your trigger foods can make a significant difference.

There is a difference between a trigger food and what motivates you to take the first bite, and the Trigger Food worksheet takes both into account. As with all change, identifying your trigger foods is a process that will most likely reveal itself over time. In Phase 3, we will delve deeper into the topics of identifying trigger foods, changing habits, and reversing emotional eating. You can revisit your Trigger Foods Worksheet as you develop your food plan, revise the foods you choose to eat, and as you continue to identify the trigger foods that sabotage your efforts.

Sample Trigger Foods Worksheet

Trigger Food Motivators	Description	My Trigger Foods
Convenience & Ultra-Processed Foods	What foods with added sugar, hidden sugar, or high natural sugar do you eat/buy because of their convenience? Examples: Pizza, Deli Sandwiches, French Fries, Canned Fruit, Pasta	Pizza Deli Sandwiches Fries Pasta
Habit	What foods with added sugar, hidden sugar, or high natural sugar do you eat out of habit? Examples: bagel or pastry for breakfast, snacks while watching TV, potatoes for dinner, crackers before bed, latte while out shopping	Breakfast: pastries Lunch: Sandwiches Dinner: Potatoes, Rice Snacks: Cheese/ Crackers
Life Situations	List 3 life situations that motivate you to eat trigger foods. What trigger foods do you eat in those situations? Examples: Holidays/Celebrations, Going Out to Eat, Office Parties	Birthday Parties: Cake Restaurants: Bread, Potatoes, Dessert Office Parties: Cookies or other sweets
HALT	What trigger foods do you eat if you let yourself become too Hungry, Angry, Lonely, or Tired?	H: Cookies, Crackers A: Cookies, Crackers, Fries L: Cookies, Chocolate T: Cookies
Emotional Eating	List 3-4 emotions that motivate you to eat trigger foods. What trigger foods do you eat when you feel these emotions?	Anxious/Stressed Afraid/Worried Depressed Bored Cookies, Cake, Chips, Ice Cream, Lattes

Trigger Foods Worksheet

Trigger Food Motivators	Description	My Trigger Foods
Convenience & Ultra-Processed Foods	What foods with added sugar, hidden sugar, or high natural sugar do you eat/buy because of their convenience?	
Habit	What foods with added sugar, hidden sugar, or high natural sugar do you eat out of habit?	Breakfast: Lunch: Dinner: Other:
Life Situations	List 3 life situations that motivate you to eat trigger foods. What trigger foods do you eat in those situations?	
HALT	What trigger foods do you eat if you let yourself become too Hungry, Angry, Lonely or Tired?	H: A: L: T:
Emotional Eating	List 3-4 emotions that motivate you to eat trigger foods. What trigger foods do you eat when you feel these emotions?	

Change Your Plate: Add in 50% Non-Starchy Vegetables

Filled with vitamins, minerals, fiber and antioxidants, fresh vegetables are critical for helping you maintain healthy blood sugar levels, avoid insulin resistance, and steer clear of roller coaster blood sugar levels. Try to include raw and lightly steamed vegetables along with other preparation methods such as stir frying and roasting vegetables. Choose as many richly colored vegetables as possible that provide needed micronutrients (vitamins and minerals) and Phytochemicals.

Micronutrients include vitamins and minerals that are essential for enabling enzymes to perform vital bodily functions, which keep us alive and healthy. Classifications include:

- Fat-Soluble Vitamins: A, D, E, K
- Water Soluble Vitamins: B Complex, C
- Major Minerals: Calcium, Phosphorus, Potassium, Sodium, Chloride, Magnesium, Sulfur
- Minor Trace Minerals: Boron, Chromium, Copper, Iodine, Iron, Manganese, Molybdenum, Selenium, Silicon, Vanadium, Zinc

Phytochemicals are nutrients found in plant foods that enhance health and help fight disease, including aiding in cell repair and acting as antioxidants to neutralize damaging free radicals. Types of phytochemicals include:

- **Flavonoids** that are found in cranberries, strawberries, apples, onions, tea, cocoa, and red wine. Studies show a link between a high intake of flavonoids and reduced risk of heart attack and stroke.
- **Carotenoids,** which are responsible for the red, orange, or yellow color of many fruits and vegetables. Their presence is masked by chlorophyll in dark green leafy vegetables.
- **Isoflavones**. Soybeans are a common source of isoflavones.

How Vitamins and Minerals Support Health

The role of vitamins and minerals is to help enzymes perform their function of catalyzing the chemical reactions that occur constantly throughout your body. If an enzyme is lacking an essential vitamin or mineral, it cannot perform properly.

The diagram below shows an example of the synergy between vitamins and enzymes.

Enzyme	Co-Enzyme	Result
Proline hydroxylase: Involved in collagen synthesis. Examples: wound healing and maintaining healthy gums.	**Vitamin C**: Enables the enzyme Proline hydroxylase to do its job in the collagen synthesis process.	Without Vitamin C, enzyme function is impaired, resulting in failure of wounds to heal, bleeding gums, and easy bruising.

Non-Starchy Vegetables

Type	Recommended Choices	Notes and Guidelines
GREEN	Alfalfa sprouts, Artichokes, Arugula, Asparagus, Broccoli, Broccolini, Bok Choy, Broccoli Rabe, Brussels Sprouts, Celery, Cucumbers, Edamame*Endive, Fennel, Green Beans, Green Bell Peppers, Green Cabbage Leafy Greens/Lettuce (Arugula Bib Lettuce, Butterhead Lettuce, Collard Greens, Dandelion Greens, Endive, Iceberg Lettuce, Kale, Mesclun, Romaine Lettuce, Parsley, Swiss Chard, Watercress) Leeks, Okra, Snow Peas, Scallions, Spinach, Watercress, Zucchini	*Edamame is also classified as a bean.
PURPLE	Eggplant, Purple Cabbage	
RED	Radicchio, Radishes, Red Okra, Red Onions, Red Peppers, Rhubarb, Tomatoes (whole and small cherry tomatoes)	
WHITE	Cauliflower, Garlic, Ginger, Hearts of Palm, Jerusalem Artichokes, Jicama, Kohlrabi, Mushrooms, Onions, Sauerkraut, Shallots, Water Chestnuts	
YELLOW & ORANGE	Carrots, Rutabagas, Yellow & Orange Bell Peppers, Yellow Summer Squash	Some consider carrots to be a "high-carb" vegetable, but they can be eaten occasionally, in moderation, unless they are a trigger food for you.
MARINE PLANTS	Seaweed (Arame, Dulse, Hijiki, Irish Moss, Kelp, Kombu, Nori, Sea Lettuce, Wakame)	Full of nutrients, various seaweeds can be included as

		part of your vegetables for the day.
FRUITS that are typically eaten as vegetables	Avocado, Hot Peppers, Olives	These foods are technically fruits, but can be included in your vegetable portion for a meal or snack.

What About Organic?

Using organic foods will help to avoid the growing list of additives that are finding their way into increasingly overly processed commercialized foods. Organic products must be produced using agricultural production practices that foster resource cycling, promote ecological balance, maintain and improve soil and water quality, minimize the use of synthetic materials, and conserve biodiversity. This section provides an overview of the key requirements and various labeling categories allowed under the USDA organic regulations, as well as the Environmental Working Group's ranking of fruits and vegetables based on their level of pesticide contamination.

You can go to www.foodnews.org to see the Environmental Working Group's latest list of fruits and vegetables and their ranking in terms of pesticide levels. If your budget is a consideration, try to purchase organic foods to replace foods that are high in pesticides.

- In 2025, among the cleanest were pineapple, sweet corn, avocados, onions, papaya, sweet peas (frozen), asparagus, cabbage, cauliflower, watermelon, mangoes, bananas, carrots, mushrooms, and kiwi.
- In 2025, the highest in pesticides were strawberries, spinach, kale, collards, mustard greens, grapes, peaches, pears, nectarines, apples, cherries, blueberries, blackberries, bell peppers, hot peppers, green beans, and potatoes.

To claim that a product is **"100 percent Organic"** (or a similar statement)

- The product must contain 100 percent organically produced ingredients (excluding salt and water, which are considered natural)

To claim that a food is **"Organic"** (or a similar statement)

- The product must contain at least 95% organic ingredients, not counting added water and salt.
- Up to 5 percent of ingredients may be nonorganic agricultural products and/or nonagricultural products on the National List (nonorganic agricultural products and several nonagricultural products on the National List may only be used if they are not commercially available as organic)

To claim that a product is **"Made with Organic Ingredients"** (or a similar statement)

- The product must contain at least 70% organic ingredients, not counting added water and salt.

To claim that a product has some organic ingredients

- Specific organic ingredients may be listed in the ingredient statement of products containing less than 70 percent organic contents—for example, "Ingredients: water, barley, beans, organic tomatoes, salt."

Tips for Eating More Non-Starchy Vegetables

- Serve raw vegetables with dip, cheese, or favorite spread
- Grill an onion
- Munch on some edamame
- Use lettuce leaves as a substitute for bread
- Munch on some celery with almond or peanut butter
- Make a tomato and onion salad
- Add onions, corn and red pepper to black beans
- Flavor up salad dressing with finely chopped veggies
- Make some salsa or pico de gallo
- Use frozen vegetables for easy side dishes
- Add vegetables to quinoa (hot or cold salad)
- Lightly steam or boil some kale
- Make a creamy soup with leftover vegetables
- Make a cucumber salad
- Make a stir fry with vegetables and protein of choice
- Prepare a batch of homemade vegetable soup
- Enjoy a bowl of vegetarian chili
- Roast a variety of Vegetables
- Press Some Red or Green Cabbage

Vitamins and Antioxidants

Everyone's biological makeup and nutritional needs are unique. Simple blood tests can reveal low levels of key vitamins/minerals such as vitamin D and magnesium. There are also newer genetic tests that can tell you what supplements may be helpful based on the presence of gene variations that influence a person's overall health.

On the following pages, you will find a list of some targeted nutritional supplements that are worth looking into. The list is not exhaustive, but it comprises some of the key vitamins, minerals, and herbal supplements that have shown promise in helping to manage blood sugar levels, as well as diabetes and its complications.

You should always consult your physician or other member of your healthcare team before adding supplements to confirm that they do not interfere with any current medications and that they do not have any harmful effects based on your specific physical condition.

Alpha Lipoic Acid	Alpha lipoic acid is a sulfur-containing compound that helps burn glucose, converting it to energy that powers your heart, brain, and other organs. Glucose is a potent generator of free radicals, which cause much of the cell damage and complications associated with diabetes. Alpha Lipoic acid is a powerful and versatile antioxidant that serves to protect the body against free radical damage. It is almost unique in that it is both water and fat soluble, enabling it to enter virtually all areas of the cells to neutralize free radicals. Alpha Lipoic Acid has been demonstrated to improve insulin sensitivity and may help diabetics by facilitating better conversion of sugar into energy. By lowering glucose levels in the bloodstream and improving insulin sensitivity, alpha lipoic acid greatly reduces a major source of free radicals. Alpha Lipoic Acid shows promise in protecting individuals against diabetic complications, including improving diabetic neuropathy. Studies have shown that it reduces the glycosylation of proteins, improves blood flow to peripheral nerves, and stimulates the regeneration of nerve fibers.

Co-Enzyme Q10	CoQ10 improves energy production in our bodies and serves as an antioxidant. These effects are especially beneficial in the prevention of heart disease and cancer. Studies also show a benefit for improved glucose control.
Vitamin C	Because insulin helps transport vitamin C into cells, diabetics are prone to having low intracellular concentrations of this vitamin, even if blood levels are normal. Vitamin C strengthens the blood vessels, especially the small capillaries, boosts the activity of the immune system, and helps protect against cardiovascular disease. Some studies suggest that vitamin C may reduce the accumulation of sorbitol in the cells, another probable cause of diabetic complications. If you are using a CGM (Continuous Glucose Monitor), you may be advised to restrict your consumption of vitamin C.
Vitamin E	Vitamin E functions primarily as an antioxidant in protecting against damage to the cell membranes. It is comprised of compounds known as tocopherols, which are needed to protect the lipids, or fats, in cell walls from damage. Vitamin E provides benefits in protecting against heart disease and strokes. Some studies suggest that vitamin E improves insulin action and exerts a number of beneficial effects that may aid in preventing long-term complications of diabetes, especially cardiovascular disease.
B Complex Vitamins	B3 is a player in many important functions, including energy production as well as the metabolism of carbohydrates and the action of insulin. Biotin helps the body metabolize carbohydrates, proteins, and fats. It is thought to help lower blood glucose levels by improving insulin sensitivity while also stimulating the activity of an enzyme called glucokinase, known to play a role in the glucose uptake by the liver. B6, B12, and Folic Acid are shown to reduce the risk of cardiovascular disease. Vitamins B6 and B12 may also be beneficial in preventing diabetic neuropathy. Folic acid has been shown to help control homocysteine levels. Although all the reasons are not fully clear, there is increasing research that shows that there is a link between high levels of homocysteine in the blood and diminished arterial health.

Vitamin D	Vitamin D regulates the absorption and use of calcium and phosphorous. New research shows it also plays a role in the regulation of normal blood sugars.

Minerals

Vanadium	Vanadium has been identified as one of the few compounds other than insulin that can activate GLUT-4 transporters, in essence mimicking the action of insulin. (Insulin stimulates GLUT-4 transporters to rise to the surface of the cell and carry glucose inside).
Chromium	Chromium has been shown to improve the activity of insulin and to facilitate the uptake of glucose into the cells. Chromium also supports carbohydrate, protein and lipid metabolism.
Magnesium	Magnesium has been shown to improve insulin production and response, thus further promoting optimal blood sugar levels. In addition to the many functions magnesium performs in our bodies, it has a relaxing effect on the smooth muscle tissues that line the arteries (resulting in improved blood flow, lower blood pressure, and a reduction in the likelihood of arterial spasms that may contribute to a heart attack). Magnesium can help decrease the risk of diabetic complications associated with arterial problems such as heart disease and retinopathy.
Calcium	In addition to helping strengthen bones, calcium may serve as a protective factor against high blood pressure.

Change Your Plate: Add in 25% Healthy Protein

Protein is an important part of your food plan. Your body requires amino acids that are genetically encoded in proteins in order to function properly. Nine of these amino acids are "essential amino acids" that can only be obtained from protein foods. The body can produce the other amino acids from the essential amino acids that you ingest from various foods. You can obtain protein from both animal and plant sources, depending upon your lifestyle and preferences. Plant sources include legumes/beans, soy products, grains, nuts, seeds, and vegetables. Typical animal protein sources are fish, poultry, eggs, dairy products, and lean meat. If you include animal protein in your food plan, closely monitor the saturated fat content.

Protein Overview and Tips for Choosing Healthy Protein

Poultry	**Best Choice**: Organic (chickens raised on organic feed with no pesticides, chemicals, or antibiotics)	If organic is not available, try to purchase poultry that is antibiotic-free (note that all chicken is hormone-free based on USDA Standards)
Beef	**Best Choice** Lean, Grass-Fed Beef	Meat from grass-fed animals contains more conjugated linoleic acid (a component of fat that boosts fat burning and the buildup of lean muscle mass) and more Omega-3 fats.
Pork	**Best Choice**: Lean Cuts **Occasional**: Ham, Bacon (Sugar Free Brands)	Consider nitrate-free brands
Fish	Wild Salmon, Sardines, Herring, Sablefish, Albacore Tuna from U.S./Canada	Try to choose fish with: High Eco Rating, low mercury content, high Omega 3 content
Shellfish & Other Seafood	Calamari, Lobster, Oysters, Mussels, Shrimp	

Eggs	**Cage Free**: Hens are able to roam vertically and horizontally in indoor spaces while having access to fresh food and water. **Free Range**: The same conditions as Cage Free with access to the outdoors during their laying cycle. **Pasture Raised**: Hens are raised with access to plants, insects, outdoor space, fresh air, & protection from the elements as needed. **Organic**: Hens are fed food free of animal byproducts, pesticides, chemical additives, or synthetic fertilizers, and they must be free to roam in their houses and have access to the outside (no antibiotics are given unless needed for infection).	NOTE: The USDA has banned the use of hormones for all hens. All eggs, even without this label are hormone free. Omega 3 Enhanced Eggs: Chickens are fed a diet of flaxseed and/or fish oils.
Dairy Products	**Milk**: the base form of all dairy products (Whole, 2%, 1%, Skim). **Cream**: Whipped, Sour, Clotted, Half and Half, Cream, Light and Crème Fraiche. **Butter**: Types include Unsalted, Salted, Sweet Cream, Cultured, Ghee, Organic, Grass-Fed, and Plant-Based. **Cheese**: Hard & Soft Cheeses **Yogurt**: Types include: Traditional, Greek, Skyre/ Icelandic, Australian, French, Lactose-Free, Dairy Alternative Yogurts. **Kefir:** A drink similar to drinkable yogurt but with a longer fermentation process. What makes kefir unique is that kefir grains are blended into the milk.	Consume dairy in moderation, and consult your physician if you have any conditions where the fat content is a concern. Dairy contains the natural sugar lactose (composed of two simpler sugars: glucose and galactose). Avoid dairy products with high amounts of lactose or added sugar. (If you are lactose intolerant, choose lactose-free dairy products.)

Legumes: Lentils & Beans	**Beans:** Adzuki, Anasazi, Black, Black-eyed peas, Borlotti, Cannellini, Chickpea, Edamame, Fava, Flageolet, Great Northern, Lima, Lupin, Kidney, Mung, Navy, Pink, Pinto, Soybeans **Lentils:** Brown, Green, Red/Yellow, French, Black Beluga	**Beans** are a great source of protein and soluble fiber. If you are concerned about phytic acid in beans, the best way to reduce the amount of phytic acid is to soak your beans overnight before cooking them. If you use canned beans, rinse them well to reduce the sodium content.
Nuts & Seeds	**Seeds**: Chia, Flax, Hemp, Pine Nuts, Pumpkin, Sesame, Sunflower **Nuts**: Almonds, Cashews, Hazelnuts, Macadamia, Pecans, Pistachios, Walnuts	
Soybeans & Products	Edamame, Tofu, Tempeh	Avoid overconsumption of highly processed soy
High Protein Grains	Wheat Berries, Teff, Amaranth, Farro, Oats, Millet, Buckwheat, Barley	Consume whole grains in moderation. Avoid highly processed grain products and all grain-based flours that cause a sharp increase in blood glucose levels and a rapid or high influx of insulin.

Quinoa	Although technically a seed, quinoa is considered a pseudocereal that is a source of protein, fiber, and carbohydrates. **Types**: Red, White, Yellow, Black	Quinoa is a gluten-free, complete protein, containing all nine essential amino acids.
High Protein Vegetables	**Non-Starchy**: Asparagus, Artichoke Hearts, Broccoli, Brussels sprouts, Cauliflower, Collard Greens, Mushrooms, Mustard Greens, Spinach **Starchy**: Green Peas, Split Peas, Sweet Corn, Sweet Potatoes,	
Protein Powder	**Animal Sources**: Whey Protein, Bone Broth, Casein, Collagen, Egg White **Plant Sources**: Hemp, Pea, Rice, Soy	Look for brands with No Added Sugar. The best whey protein powder is free of bovine growth hormones, preferably whey protein isolate or a combo of whey protein concentrate and isolate. (isolate contains more protein with less fat and lactose per serving)

Change Your Plate: Add a 25% Combo of Healthy Fats and Quality Carbohydrates.

In moderation, it is important to include certain "good for you" fats in your food plan. Among other things, fats are required for hormone production, facilitation of oxygen transport and calcium absorption, and for the absorption of the fat-soluble vitamins A, D, E, and K.

Fats are made up of building blocks called fatty acids. The structure of the fat molecule determines whether a fat is considered saturated or unsaturated. There are two types of unsaturated fats in the foods that we eat: Polyunsaturated fats and Monounsaturated Fats. These are shown in the chart below:

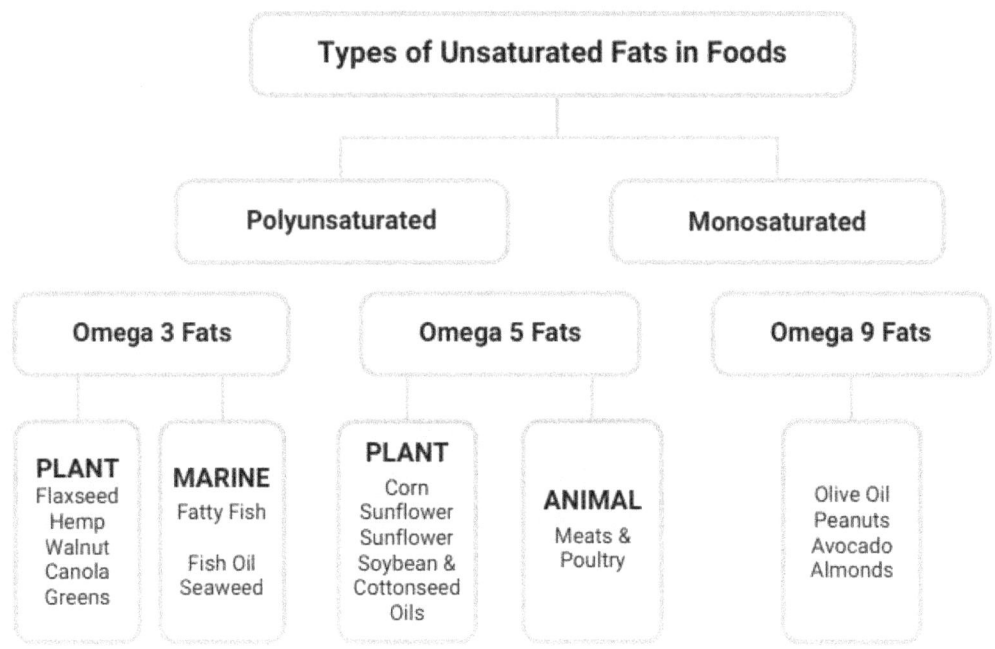

Essential Fatty Acids Overview

EFA's (generally)	Essential fatty acids are a type of fatty acid that cannot be produced in the body and must be obtained through diet or supplementation. Following ingestion, EFA's are ultimately converted to substances called prostaglandins that act like hormones to help regulate a myriad of physiological functions, including cardiovascular health and fat metabolism. EFAs come in two common classes: Omega-3's and Omega 6's.
Omega 3	Three essential fatty acids are found in omega-3 fats and oils: alpha-linoleic acid, eicosatetraenoic acid (EPA), and Docosahexaenoic acid (DHA). Omega 3's provide a number of benefits including: relaxing constricted arteries, repairing tissue damage caused by clogged arteries, reducing levels of VLDSs (very low-density lipoproteins, which are clusters of lipids linked to heart disease), lowering the rate at which the liver makes triglycerides, and stabilizing heart cells, making them more resistant to irregular beats that can cause heart attacks.

Omega 6	The most important of the omega-6 fatty acids for the diabetic is gamma linolenic acid (GLA). This fatty acid is derived from the EFA linolenic acid. You can get linoleic acid from vegetables, nuts, and seed oils, but many diabetics are deficient in GLA because they often have problems converting the linolenic acid to GLA. Without the enzyme delta-6-desaturase (D6D), omega-6's won't transform into GLA. We lose D6D as we grow older, and it is suppressed by a diet including a lot of sugar, alcohol, margarine, or other partially hydrogenated oils. Supplemental GLA may be helpful in helping to improve peripheral neuropathy, which is caused by inflammation and deterioration of the peripheral nerves, usually in the legs and feet. Sources of GLA include evening primrose and borage oil.
Nattokinase	An enzyme that has been shown to promote healthy circulation and reduce the risk of blood clots.

- Omega 3 Fats and Omega 6 fats have opposite effects in the body. Omega 6 fats impede the benefits of Omega 3 fats, and if these two fats are not properly balanced in your diet, the overload of Omega 6 fats can dramatically affect your health.

- Omega 3 fats fight inflammation and keep blood vessels healthy by decreasing blood pressure and triglycerides, keeping arteries flexible and wide for smooth blood flow, and decreasing clotting and clumping of blood cells. Additionally, Omega 3 fats keep brain cell membranes healthy and fluid. Omega 3 fats from plant sources differ from Omega 3 fatty acids found in seafood. Plant sources contain ALA, which is known as a "short chain" "fatty acid" that can be turned into EPA and DHA. These are the two longer chain fatty acids that provide the many powerhouse benefits of Omega 3 fats.

- High amounts of Omega 6 fats increase inflammation, blood clotting, and insulin resistance. For optimal health try to limit the consumption of Omega 6 fats and increase your intake of Omega 3 fats. Most dietary Omega 6 fats come from salad dressings, cooking oils, and spreads. One way to decrease your consumption of Omega 6 fats is to eat more monounsaturated fats, which have no negative effect on Omega-3 fats and also lower cholesterol. Olive oil is the

lowest in omega-6 fats. In moderation, nuts and avocados are also excellent sources of healthy fats.
- Limit the amount of saturated fats in your diet. Saturated fat raises levels of LDL cholesterol and increases the risk of heart disease. Depending on your condition, you can include small amounts of certain saturated fats in your food plan (such as organic butter from grass-fed cows, coconut butter, Ghee, and certain cheeses). But always discuss this with your physician if you have a serious diabetic complication, such as heart disease.
- The only fats that should be totally avoided are trans fatty acids. These are chemically altered vegetable oils that typically show up in foods as hydrogenated or partially hydrogenated oil. Trans fatty acids are commonly found in margarine, peanut butter, commercial snacks, baked goods, and fried foods. These fats increase the risk of heart disease to a greater degree than saturated fats because, in addition to raising total cholesterol, they lower protective HDL cholesterol. Growing research indicates that trans fats are connected not only to cancer, heart disease, and aging, but also to immune system suppression and diminished ability to utilize essential fatty acids. Read labels carefully, and always choose products that don't contain these damaging fats.

Increase Fiber

Fiber provides tremendous benefits, including managing blood sugar levels. Remember to start adding fiber to your diet slowly to avoid gas/bloating and build up to 20 to 30 grams daily. Fiber is the part of food that cannot be digested or broken down into a form of energy for our body. It is considered a type of complex carbohydrate, but it cannot be absorbed to produce energy. Fiber comes only from plants, fruits, vegetables, nuts, seeds, and grains. No animal products contain fiber.

Fiber comes in two forms: insoluble and soluble fiber. While we need both types each day, soluble fiber appears to play an especially important role in glucose control. This is because it forms a thick gel that interferes with the absorption of glucose in the intestine, thereby reducing the ups and downs of blood sugar levels.

It also helps to bind cholesterol in the intestinal tract, which is why it may help to lower cholesterol levels.

	Soluble Fiber	Insoluble Fiber
DEFINED	Technically called pectin, gum, and mucilage, soluble fiber dissolves and breaks down in water, forming a thick gel.	Technically called cellulose, hemicellulose, and lignin, insoluble fiber does not dissolve in water or break down in your digestive system.
FUNCTIONS	Prolongs stomach emptying time so that sugar is released and absorbed more slowly. Binds with fatty acids, which are the building blocks of fat.	Moves bulk through the intestines. Controls and balances the PH (i.e., degree of acidity or alkalinity) in the intestines.
BENEFITS	Helps to regulate blood sugar levels, lower cholesterol, and remove toxins from your body. Slows the absorption of food after meals, slowing down the conversion of carbohydrates to sugar. This allows glucose to be burned more efficiently, rather than being stored as fat.	Promotes regular bowel movements and prevents constipation. Removes toxic waste from the colon. Helps prevent colon cancer by keeping an optimal pH in the intestines to prevent microbes from producing cancerous substances.
SOURCES	Soluble fiber is abundant in beans, oats, barley, fruits, and many vegetables.	Insoluble fiber is the roughage found in vegetables and the skins and outer coatings of grains, fruits, and legumes.

In addition to helping regulate blood sugar levels, fiber-rich foods tend to be lower in calories and can also help curb appetite. A hormone, Cholecystokinin (CCK), released by cells in the small intestine, signals the brain to feel full and satisfied. The combination of nutrients and fiber from foods such as beans plays a role in enhancing CCK effects and overall satisfaction from food.

The easiest way to ensure you get enough fiber in your diet is to eat a wide variety of foods centered around a diet rich in high-fiber, nutrient-dense vegetables, low-glycemic-index fruits, and healthy protein. In addition to vegetables, some good sources of fiber include:

- **Flax**. Always grind flax seeds before eating. You can grind your own or purchase ground flax seeds. Ground flax can be added to recipes, sprinkled on yogurt and salads, or included in your favorite smoothly.
- **Nuts**. If you don't have any nut allergies, include a few handfuls of almonds, walnuts, pecans, or hazelnuts in your diet every day.
- **Legumes**. Beans have high soluble fiber content and can be consumed in numerous ways. Enjoy them in salads, as side dishes, or in your favorite chili recipe, and there are just a few ways to incorporate beans into your food plan.

Stay Hydrated.

Do you ever feel hungry soon after eating or tired when you know you have had a good night's sleep? Guess what? You may be dehydrated. Often, drinking a glass of water when you have these symptoms will relieve the tiredness or feeling of hunger. Other signs of dehydration include constipation or dark urine.

Water is essential for the proper functioning of every cell in your body and provides a number of important functions, from lubricating joints, transporting nutrients to your muscles, and carrying away waste such as carbon dioxide and lactic acid. If you have diabetes, when you don't drink enough water, the glucose in your bloodstream becomes more concentrated, which leads to higher blood sugar levels.

Drinking water as your main source of liquid is conducive to a healthy lifestyle because your body is largely made up of water, and it is necessary for healthy body functions. While it's true that, for most people, plain water is the best thing to drink to stay hydrated, there are plenty of alternative beverage options if you don't like the taste of plain water or want some variety. You can also get water into your system from food sources, such as soup, fruits, and vegetables that contain a high percentage of water.

How Much Water is Enough?

Although many experts recommend drinking six to eight 8-ounce glasses of water or other liquids each day, this is more of a guideline than an exact requirement. Your actual hydration needs will depend upon the climate where you live, your age, and your physical condition. People who live in hot climates or who exercise frequently often need more water than more sedentary individuals who live in temperate places. Most healthy people can stay hydrated by following their bodies' cues and drinking when thirsty.

Common signs of dehydration include fatigue, headaches, nausea, and dizziness. Your best defense against dehydration is to become conscious of drinking liquids throughout the day and including some foods with a high percentage of water in your daily food plan.

If you are not sure how much liquid you should be consuming, discuss this with your physician. He or she can help you determine the amount of water that's right for you. If you are under a physician's care for congestive heart failure, vascular disease, lung disease, or renal disease, increasing your fluid intake should not be attempted without consulting your physician.

Avoid Soda (including Diet) and Fruit Juice

Both soda and fruit juice contain way too much sugar. Additionally, a growing body of research indicates that drinking artificially sweetened diet sodas on a regular basis may set you up for weight gain and increased cravings for sweets. Artificially sweetened sodas can also interfere with your body's signal to tell you to stop eating. An occasional diet soda, such as when you are eating out, is probably OK, unless it is a trigger food for you.

What About Drinking Tea?

When I delved into research on the topic of hydration, I found various opinions on whether part of your hydration needs can be met with tea.

The pros of this option are the many established health benefits, including heart-protecting and disease-annihilating antioxidants. The cons mainly centered around the debate concerning whether the caffeine in black, green, white, and oolong tea makes it a poor choice for hydration.

For those of you who like to drink tea, the good news is that newer studies are finding that the benefits of tea outweigh any effects of the caffeine, and that when consumed in moderation (2-3 small to medium cups per day) there is no significant dehydrating effect from the caffeine (There are also many brands that make decaffeinated options).

Most people are familiar with black, oolong, green, and white teas. But there are many different healthy tea options.

- Black tea and oolong tea leaves undergo the most processing, that includes a crushing and fermentation process.
- Green tea leaves are not fermented, they are withered and steamed. Green tea is produced from leaves that have not withered or oxidized.
- White tea comes from young leaves and buds. White tea is the least processed of all teas and has a sweeter, milder flavor than green tea.
- Another type of tea, Rooibos (pronounced ROY-boss) (also referred to as Red Tea), comes from a different plant, and unlike the teas above, it does not contain any caffeine.
- Other herbal choices include teas like chamomile, peppermint, and lavender.

Another type of tea that most people don't know about is an all-natural tea brewed from vegetables. For a relaxing, energizing tea that also quiets sugar cravings, try the following sweet vegetable tea.

Bring 3 cups of water to a boil, then lower the heat and add ¼ cup of onions, ¼ cup of carrots, ¼ cup of cabbage, and ¼ cup of either parsnips or butternut squash. The vegetables should be cut into small chunks. Simmer covered for 15-20 minutes. Strain the tea, discard the vegetables, and then pour the liquid into a cup, and enjoy.

Hydration Tips and Ideas

- Strawberries, orange slices, lemons, limes, blueberries, watermelon, cucumbers, and mint are delicious options for flavoring water.
- If you are drinking a lot of iced tea, try making your own with decaf teabags.
- Set a large glass of water by the bed when you go to sleep and drink it first thing when you wake up in the morning. This pulls out toxins left from the previous day and refreshens your system, preparing it for the day ahead.

- Keep water accessible throughout the day, whether you're on the go or sitting at a desk. Having water close by will remind you to take a sip when thirsty. The first sip of water will usually let you know how much you need.
- If you have most of your water before early evening, the possibility of interrupted sleep will not be an issue because you will not crave a big glass before bed.
- A cup of hot chamomile tea at night is a relaxing way to end your day.
- You can also get water into your system from food sources, such as soups and vegetables that contain a high percentage of water.

Create Your 7 Day Meal Plan

	Breakfast	Lunch	Dinner
Day 1			
Day 2			
Day 3			
Day 4			
Day 5			

	Breakfast	Lunch	Dinner
Day 6			
Day 7			

Adopt New Habits: Watch Portion Sizes

One serving is approximately equivalent to:

Fruit & Vegetables	Whole Grains
• ½ cup cooked or raw veggies • 1 cup salad • 1 medium piece of fruit • ½ chopped fruit • ¾ cup vegetable juice	• 1 slice of bread • ½ cup cooked grain or pasta • ½ -1 cup dry cereal • 3-4 crackers
Protein Foods	**Dairy**
• ½ cup cooked beans • 1 whole egg, 3 egg whites, or 2 egg whites with one yolk • 2-3 oz. Meat, Fish, or Poultry (approx. size of deck of cards) • 4 oz. Tofu, ½ cup soy milk, ½ cup soy protein • ¾ cup vegetable or fruit juice	• 1 cup milk • 4 oz. Cheese (4 cubes) • ½ cup cottage cheese or part-skim ricotta • 1 cup yogurt
	Fats, Nuts & Seeds
	• 1 TBSP oil • 2 TBSP nuts, seeds, or nut butters

Adopt New Habits: Eat Mindfully

Mindfulness is a mental state achieved when you focus your awareness on the present moment while noticing and accepting your feelings, thoughts, and bodily sensations without judgment.

Eating mindfully helps you make a connection with your food by breaking mindless routines, such as eating in front of the TV, eating while multitasking, or eating when you're bored. When you eat mindlessly, you are barely aware of what you are consuming, and this can lead to overeating and difficulties with portion control. In this state, you are moving on to the next bite before you have experienced the bite that you have in your mouth.

When you slow down enough to taste and enjoy food, you:

- Begin to enjoy what you eat,
- Eat less, and
- Make better decisions about what to eat.

Tips for Mindful Eating

Heighten your awareness of what you are eating: This means slowing down when you eat, paying attention to what you are eating, and really tasting and enjoying your food.

Become aware of mindless eating: Here are some common reasons that people engage in mindless eating. Be aware if any of these apply when you are eating food. Don't beat yourself up if you find yourself eating for reasons other than hunger; becoming aware is a first step towards changing habitual eating habits.

- To relieve boredom or stress
- To find comfort in tough situations
- To quiet negative thoughts or to numb emotions
- Out of habit (example: to use food as a reward or to eat while watching TV)
- To navigate social situations (such as mindlessly eating at a party when you aren't really hungry)

- Stop or limit multitasking when you eat. Giving your food your complete attention enables you to connect with your body and supports eating out of hunger, not to feed your emotions.

Mindful Eating Exercise

In this exercise, you are going to explore slowing down to enjoy the actual experience of eating either a small piece of sugar-free dark chocolate, a ripe strawberry, a spoonful of nut butter, or another type of ripe fruit (or, if these are trigger foods for you, a piece of cooked vegetable of choice) (I don't recommend using a raw vegetable or anything crunchy for this exercise and it should be something that you like to eat).

FIRST, take a minute to understand how you typically consume food. What is your state of mind when eating?

- Most often, I am mindlessly unaware, multi-tasking when eating, and unaware of portion sizes (for example, eating directly out of a bag or standing in front of the refrigerator, eating).
- Most often, I am eating rapidly, taking big bites, and I tend to finish everything on my plate.
- Most often, I am very inattentive to what I am eating, not really tasting the food.
- Sometimes I am aware of portion sizes. Occasionally, I notice the taste, texture, and smell of my food.
- Sometimes, I am alert. For 25% of my eating experience, I chew my food several times, and my attention is directed to eating.
- I make a conscious effort to be mindfully aware when I eat. I chew at least 25 times when I eat, or at the very least, I am aware of every bite and fully chew it before swallowing.
- I pay attention to the sensations of the food I am eating. I enjoy every bite.

When you are ready, select the food for your Mindful Eating Exercise, place it on a small plate, and move through the steps below in a quiet space. Make sure to turn off your phone and remove yourself from any other distractions.

What does the food you chose look like? How food looks is one of the first things that either attracts or repels us from a food, and makes us want to eat more or less of it. Imagine you are a Martian scientist. You just arrived on Earth and have never seen this food before. Look at it carefully. What does the essence of the food bring to mind? Do you have a pleasant or negative reaction to this food? Is your reaction because of what the food actually looks like or something else?

Experience the aroma. The aroma of food has a lot to do with our enjoyment of that food. Bring the food up to your nose. Experience smelling the food, and then describe what you smell. Is it a pleasant or negative experience? Notice what thoughts come into your mind as you do this. The smell of a certain food can bring up some powerful feelings and memories. Deeply Inhale. Do any critical thoughts come up like, "I shouldn't eat this?" If so, let the thoughts come and go as if you are letting go of a balloon.

How does the food feel in your mouth? Slowly take a small bite of the food (YES, do not put the whole piece of chocolate, or whatever food you chose, in your mouth at one time…). Don't chew or swallow it yet, just let it sit on your tongue and for a moment become aware of the taste and sensations of the food on your tongue. How does it feel and taste as it releases its flavors to your taste buds?

Experience the flavor and texture before chewing. Very slowly, swirl the food around to savor it for a moment in your mouth. What is the flavor sensation? Sweet? Bitter? What about the texture? Smooth? Creamy? There are hundreds of words to describe the experience of tasting. Try to notice the moment when you feel like you want to chew and swallow. Then, slowly chew and then swallow the chocolate (or other food chosen), focusing on the sensations as it disappears from your mouth and noticing any lingering tastes or sensations.

Continue eating the food in tiny bites until it is finished. What came to mind as you were eating it? Were you "bored," eager to finish, or was eating mindfully a new but interesting or good experience? Do you want more? If yes, is your appetite really hungry for more, sort of wanting it, or do you feel like you have had enough? Having a second piece or a spoonful of the food you chose is fine.

Repeat the exercise until the piece of food you chose is gone. If you find that you still want more after your second helping, stop and take some deep breaths or just close your eyes and relax for a moment. Have a cup of water or hot tea and see how you feel after.

The next time you are eating a snack or meal, remember this exercise and consciously slow down to experience and enjoy your food.

Adopt New Habits: Be Aware of Your Eating Schedule and Avoid Nighttime Eating

Do You Experience Night-Time Eating?

Do you ever find yourself eating way past dinner, often with multiple snacks throughout the evening? For many, this could just be a habit that can be broken with some basic behavioral changes. But, based on new studies, repetitive nighttime eating can be an actual eating disorder called Night Eating Syndrome.

- People with NES feel very hungry after dinner and tend to graze on snacks repeatedly at night.
- They may wake up from sleep feeling a strong urge to eat. It may also feel like they can't go back to sleep without eating.
- NES is more common in people with diabetes or who are overweight, which may be related to disturbed sleep patterns and altered metabolism.
- NES is also often associated with insomnia because people with NES feel so hungry at night, they have trouble getting to sleep, wake up at night to eat, or can't go back to sleep without eating.
- A history of depression, anxiety, and substance abuse are also more common in people with NES.

- Sleep troubles that come with NES also may contribute to weight gain and/or difficulty losing weight. It might also make it more difficult to manage blood sugar levels.

Possible Causes of Night Eating Syndrome

The exact cause of night eating syndrome and its link to addiction and depression is not clear. There may be a number of contributing factors leading to NES.

- One theory is that night eating syndrome involves a disruption in the hormones that regulate sleep, appetite, and mood--specifically, an alteration or disruption in the hypothalamic pituitary-adrenal axis.
- It is possible that night eating syndrome may be a form of "self-medication," since a large proportion of snacking late at night generally involves carbohydrate-rich or "comfort" type foods.
- Those with night eating syndrome may also be high achievers who work through lunch, and may then make up the caloric debt by eating more at night.
- Night eating syndrome can also be viewed as a response to dieting. With the restriction of calories during the day, people typically overcompensate at night by eating greater amounts.
- Night eating may also be a response to stress bottled up during the day, with eating serving as a way to self-medicate, according to some people with the syndrome.

Is Nighttime Eating an Occasional Habit or a More Serious Health Issue?

The first thing is to evaluate your situation to determine whether this is an ongoing issue that could negatively affect your overall health or just an occasional "situational" occurrence of wanting a snack in the evening.

If the characteristics listed below resonate with you, it may be a sign of Night Eating Syndrome. (NOTE: most nighttime eating in this category occurs when you are awake---there is a related condition characterized by sleep eating, which is different)

Below is a summary of the key characteristics of Night Time Eating Syndrome:

- At least 25% of your food intake is eaten at night, i.e., dinner and beyond (It could also start with very late afternoon snacking very close to dinnertime).
- It may take the form of grazing in small amounts throughout the evening (it does not have to involve binging on large quantities of food eaten at one or more meals or snacks).
- You often skip breakfast and/or are not very hungry throughout the day, preferring to eat late afternoon, dinner, and beyond.
- 2-3 nights a week, you wake up from sleeping to eat and feel like you won't be able to sleep unless you eat something.
- You often eat to ease anxiety or to self-soothe at night.
- Along with night eating, you experience anxiety or depression throughout the day and/or night.
- You feel unable to stop and out of control when you eat at night.
- You have interrupted sleep or insomnia several nights per week.

If you experience any of these symptoms, Night Eating Syndrome may be a contributing factor. The good news is that there are many ways to conquer nighttime eating, with the solutions differing depending on your particular underlying causes.

Gain Clarity Around Your Nighttime Eating by Answering the Questions Below

The questions are designed to help you gain more clarity and awareness around your nighttime eating and to give you the opportunity to take the next steps. This is not a diagnosis or diagnostic test and does not replace medical care.

My strong suggestion is that you use your new knowledge to start to address your night eating patterns and improve the habits that impact your night eating. If you have concerns, speak with your physician or other member of your healthcare team.

- Do you eat in the evening, especially after dinner?
- Is at least 25% of your food intake eaten at night? (either dinner and beyond or late afternoon and beyond).
- When does your nighttime eating start and end?
- Can your night eating be described as grazing and eating small amounts of different foods throughout the evening?

- In the evening hours after dinner do you binge eat?
- Do you crave sweets and carbs in the evening?
- Do you eat to ease anxiety or self sooth?
- Do you eat at night even though you're not hungry?
- Do you eat at night out of boredom?
- Do you eat carbs when you are tired or when you want to stay awake?
- Do you wake up during the night and eat? Do you recall waking up and eating?
- Do you experience insomnia four or five nights a week?
- Do you believe that eating is necessary to get to sleep or get back to sleep?
- Do you often skip breakfast?
- Are you not very hungry throughout the day, preferring to eat late afternoon, dinner, and beyond?
- Do you often have feelings of sadness, stress, anxiety, or depression?
- Do feelings of sadness, stress, or anxiety trigger eating?
- If you have depression, does your depressed mood get worse during evening hours?
- Are you experiencing weight gain?
- Are your blood sugar levels higher in the morning, and does this differ after a period of night eating as opposed to no night eating?

If you answered yes to several questions, this could be an indication of Night Eating Syndrome, which you can explore further with your healthcare team. As I noted, many nighttime eating issues can be addressed by changes in behavior and habits that can include changing daytime eating patterns, making your snacks and meals more blood sugar-friendly, and changing evening routines. If you have an eating disorder or you suspect you have issues of trauma or Night Eating Syndrome that require counseling, speak to your physician, who can refer you to the appropriate resources.

Adopt New Habits: Snack Smart

There are many different expert opinions about including snacks in your daily Food Plan. When I am practicing Intermittent Fasting, my routine is 2 meals plus a snack around 3 pm. It all depends on your biochemistry, lifestyle, and how snacks affect your ability to stay on track with your food plan. Some guidelines for snacking include:

- Snacks should be planned and eaten on a plate. Do not eat snacks out of a box or bag, and always prepare a single serving of whatever you are including in your snack.
- Your snack should never include trigger foods. If you find yourself going back for more or have cravings after eating a snack, reevaluate your snack choice.
- Do not graze. Sit down and eat your snack mindfully, even if it is a small portion.
- If you are diabetic and trying a snack food for the first time, measure your blood sugar levels after consuming your snack. If it is too high one or two hours after consumption, eliminate the snack and choose something else.

Below are some snack ideas:

- Pumpkin Seed Mix (1/4 cup) (pumpkin seeds, sunflower seeds, chopped pecans or walnuts (optional mini sugar-free chocolate chips)
- ¼ cup nuts (almonds, walnuts, pecans) with a slice of low-fat cheese or raw veggies.1 TBSP almond butter with a piece of non-grain-based bread or apple slices
- Edamame with flavored "salts," Gomashio, or Ponzu Sauce
- Turkey rollups with avocado
- Chopped salad with beans, diced tomatoes, red onions, avocado, and dressing of choice
- Cherry tomatoes with tuna or chicken salad
- Deviled egg (if desired, with hummus substituted for mashed egg yolk)
- Hummus or Bean Dip with raw vegetables
- ¼ cup part-skim ricotta cheese (or Greek Yogurt) with unsweetened cocoa and a tablespoon of chocolate protein powder. (Add Stevia or Truvia to taste). To make it extra luxurious, swirl in some melted Sugar Free Dark Chocolate.
- Cucumber or zucchini rounds with hummus, smoked salmon/cream cheese, or tuna salad
- Air Fried Chicken Strips with "no-grain-based flour coating"
- Spicy, Roasted Chickpeas

- Guacamole with Jicama sticks
- Cup of bone broth (some popular brands are Kettle & Fire, Brodo, Bare Bones, Kitchen Basics, and Pacific Foods) or soup (vegetable, lentil, bean soups with a combo of protein and vegetables)
- Sardine salad with cucumbers & vegetables
- Simple Cucumber Salad (optional add diced tomato and slices of onion)
- Homemade low carb crackers or Triscuits with smoked salmon & cream cheese
- Baby spinach "rollups" with Laughing Cow Cheese and walnuts
- Avocado Slices with lemon or lime
- Silver Dollar "no grain-based flour" Pancakes
- Mini Chaffle Pizza (add some pepperoni or vegetables on top)
- Antipasto platter (olives, roasted peppers, hummus, pickled vegetables, cheese)
- Protein Smoothie (Low glycemic fruit only)
- Small Mezze plate with a combo of protein, cheese, and vegetables
- A small serving of marinated olives with hummus
- Cooked shrimp with cocktail sauce
- Marinated vegetables
- Air fried zucchini rounds
- Artichoke Hearts

Adopt New Habits: Build a Better Breakfast

Everyone's biochemistry is different, and there is no definitive answer to the question, what should I eat for breakfast? Having said that, the best breakfast foods are those that do not cause huge blood sugar spikes, set the stage for balanced blood sugars the rest of the day, and leave you feeling satisfied. As a rule of thumb, the more nutritionally dense the foods are the better you will feel. If you are doing "intermittent fasting" you can break your fast at the appropriate time with any of the breakfast foods below.

Below are some ideas for "breaking your fast."

- Eggs or tofu scrambled with vegetables of choice. (TIP: keep some sautéed onions in the fridge. In the morning, toss them into scrambled eggs or tofu. For added flavor, add chopped peppers, broccoli, or sun-dried tomatoes.

- Choco-Greens Powder Smoothie or Very Berry Smoothie
- Hard-boiled or deviled eggs (if desired, substitute hummus for mashed egg yolk)
- Crust-free mini quiche (with vegetables and cheese of choice)
- Yogurt with protein powder, berries, and chopped nuts
- Almond butter/ricotta spread ½ sprouted whole grain English Muffin, Minute Keto English Muffin, or a piece of Keto/low-carb bread. To make the spread, combine 1 TBSP Almond Butter with ¼ cup part-skim ricotta cheese and sweeten with a sugar alternative of your choice (Add some protein powder or ground flax seed for extra nutrients).
- Turkey breast rollup with low-fat cheese, avocado, and sprouts
- Non-Grain-Based French Toast or pancakes with blueberries, or Easy Blueberry Syrup
- Breakfast Chaffles
- Almond flour or other grain-based flour protein pancakes (make your own pancakes or start with a mix). For extra protein, mix in some ricotta cheese.
- Smoked salmon, low-fat veggie cream cheese, onion, and tomato on non-grain-based bread or sprouted whole grain bread
- Poached salmon with cucumber salad
- Avocado Toast on Keto/low carb Toast or Hummus, avocado, red onion, and tomato on non-grain-based bread or sprouted whole grain English Muffin
- Egg in the Hole made with Keto/low-carb bread
- Regular Size or Mini Egg Muffins (combo of eggs, cheese, veggies, and/or breakfast meat of choice baked in muffin tin)
- Tempeh or Turkey Bacon with eggs of choice and side salad
- Bone Broth, Miso Soup or other broth (with some vegetables and/or some protein like tofu or shredded chicken added in) Some popular brands are Kettle & Fire, Brodo, Bare Bones, Kitchen Basics, and Pacific Foods.
- Swedish Breakfast Plate

Adopt New Habits to Make Food Prep Easier

One of the things I hear from members and my clients is, "I know what I need to do; I just don't have the time." Can anyone relate? If you are trying to eat better and feeling stressed, sometimes cooking is one of the first things people let go of. Unfortunately, self-care does take some time. There is no way around it, but here are some tips to make it easier.

- **Use the "almost from scratch method" to prepare meals and snacks and keep a well-stocked pantry**. This is my go-to way to stay sane. Things I always keep on hand to make quick meals and snacks include rotisserie chicken, sugar-free sauces and marinades, low carb wraps, canned artichoke hearts, canned beans, frozen veggies, good quality cheese, cooked quinoa in pouches, baked tofu, chicken and vegetable broth, olives, hummus and other healthy dips, pre-cut veggies etc. Having a well-stocked pantry of items that don't have to be cooked from scratch makes it easy to shave time off preparing meals and snacks.
- **Make mini cheese/charcuterie/mezze plates**. There are many nights I just don't feel like cooking. Putting together a beautiful plate that is a combo of foods I have on hand solves the problem and provides a visually appealing and satisfying meal. I often do themes such as 1) Italian with a plate of meats, cheeses, olives, peppers, and dips 2) Greek with hummus, tabbouleh, olives, feta cheese, and salad 3) Japanese with deconstructed sushi and cauliflower rice or 4) Mexican with beans, guacamole, lettuce, and tomatoes. You get the idea.
- **Prep ahead**. Doing some prep one day a week makes it even easier to do tips 1 & 2 above. I usually take 1 or 2 hours on a Saturday to do things like prepare pickled onions for salads, caramelize onions for stir fries/omelets or quinoa dishes, cook a pot of quinoa, cut up veggies, and make a pot of soup, stew, or meatballs that can be used throughout the week. Nothing feels better than having some pre-cooked food when you are in a hurry and hungry.
- **Have the ingredients for one or two "GO TO" options that you can eat when all else fails**. I always have the makings for a filling protein-based smoothie. There have been many nights when I could not figure out what I wanted to eat, and I prepared a filling smoothie and half of a low-carb wrap of some sort.

- **Finally, KEEP IT SIMPLE.** A beautifully put-together plate of simple foods is hugely satisfying when eaten slowly and mindfully.

Takeaways & Highlights

Putting Your Food Plan into Action

- **Get support.** You have many options, including working with a health counselor, health coach, dietitian, trainer, joining a support group, or just teaming up with a friend. (A word of caution: Be wary of fad diets or programs that are hard to follow and don't meet your long-term objectives.)
- **Take the Veggie Challenge.** Do you know how many servings of vegetables you eat in a day? A week? Use a daily journal and note how many vegetables you consume in a day or a seven-day time period. The results might surprise you.
- **Start keeping a daily food journal.** Keeping a food journal will help you to get a handle on what you are "really" eating throughout the day and allow you to observe both your food choices and patterns of eating that affect your blood sugars.
- **Each week, select a vegetable that you don't eat regularly and add it to one of your meals.** Good choices include: asparagus, broccoli, Brussels sprouts, cabbage, cauliflower, celery, collard greens, cucumber, kale, onions, green and red peppers, tomatoes, zucchini, and carrots (note: although carrots are higher on the glycemic index, they are a good source of nutrients and OK in moderation).
- **Limit your intake of "starchy" vegetables, particularly white potatoes.** Sweet potatoes, yams, peas, turnips, and corn are good sources of nutrients when eaten on occasion and in small portions.

- **Stay hydrated, stop adding sugar to beverages, and eliminate soda**: Water is the best beverage for staying hydrated. It can be "jazzed up" with infusions of fruit or vegetables such as cucumber. Tea is also a good choice, and if you are concerned about caffeine, many companies offer decaffeinated brands.
- **Avoid Diet Soda**. Many studies show that consuming diet soda can set off cravings for sweets and that drinking diet soda makes it harder to keep blood sugar levels under control.
- **Become familiar with the different types of sweeteners**. Experiment with alternative sweeteners to determine whether they are an option or whether you need to avoid them totally. If they are not a trigger food for you, there are a variety of monk fruit and Stevia liquid-flavored drops that work well in beverages.
- **Take an action step each day to avoid added sugar**. Do this regularly until you are comfortable with your sugar-free lifestyle.
- **Eliminate Grain-based flour products**. The next time you want to have a sandwich, try Sprouted Grain or a non-grain-based bread made with nut, bean, golden flaxseed, or coconut flour (or a combination of any of these flours). Skip the bread and try using a lettuce wrap, or instead create a salad with your sandwich ingredients.
- **Try substitutions for rice**. The next time you plan to eat rice, try quinoa or "cauliflower rice."
- **Try something different for breakfast**. There are no set rules for what to eat for breakfast. The key is to start the day with a satisfying breakfast that does not cause a sharp rise in blood sugars, setting the stage for healthy eating throughout the rest of the day.
- **Experiment with different protein and healthy fat options**. Both protein and healthy fats promote satiety and help to control blood sugar levels. Try different protein options and cooking methods based on your eating style (carnivorous, pescatarian, vegetarian, vegan). You can incorporate healthy fats into various dishes, such as salad dressings, marinades, or as additions to salads and recipes.
- **Bring healthy snacks to work**. The work environment is stressful, and that 3 p.m. "gotta have a snack" craving will get you every time if you are not prepared. Nut and seed mixes, low-fat cheese, almond butter with a slice of non-

grain-based bread, a cup of bone broth, or vegetables with dip are all good alternatives to the vending machine.

- **Keep a well-stocked pantry**. Being prepared is the best way to avoid turning to trigger foods when you are hungry or preparing a meal. People always ask me what I keep in my refrigerator, freezer, and pantry. Use the lists provided in this chapter as a starting point to fill your refrigerator, freezer, and pantry with foods that support your sugar-free lifestyle. In Chapter 17 (Eliminate Clutter in Your Space to Create an Environment that Supports Lasting Change) I will lead you through your own Kitchen & Pantry Makeover and share a list of recommendations and items that I keep on hand for fast and easy food preparation.

CHAPTER 13
Validate, Monitor, and Adjust Your Plan

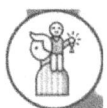

Coach on Your Shoulder

Using a Daily Journal to Stay on Track

Forming a new habit takes about 21 days of consistent action, and then it typically takes at least 90 days for new habits to become part of your daily routine. For most people, it takes about a year to make lasting lifestyle changes. It is not unusual to have setbacks in the beginning or to experience times when your results are not what you expected.

Through counseling clients, I have learned that most of us know what we need to do to achieve health goals. The difficulty comes with sticking to new behaviors when life gets in the way. A common reason that people struggle with maintaining a sugar-free lifestyle is that they don't track their progress on a daily basis, and their plans are not in sync with their unique biochemistry and goals. This can lead to frustration and, worse, quitting.

At times when you feel out of control, monitoring and adjusting your action plan can be the difference between struggling to stay on track and feeling focused and empowered to keep moving forward.

In the business world, companies engage in carefully orchestrated planning processes to navigate change and to ensure success. While managing change in our personal life does not need to be as rigorous, there are processes that are beneficial in both contexts, including:

- Strategic planning (identifying where you are now and where you want to go),
- Tactical planning (determining how you are going to get there),
- Implementation (your action steps), and
- Validation (monitoring daily activities and making adjustments as needed)

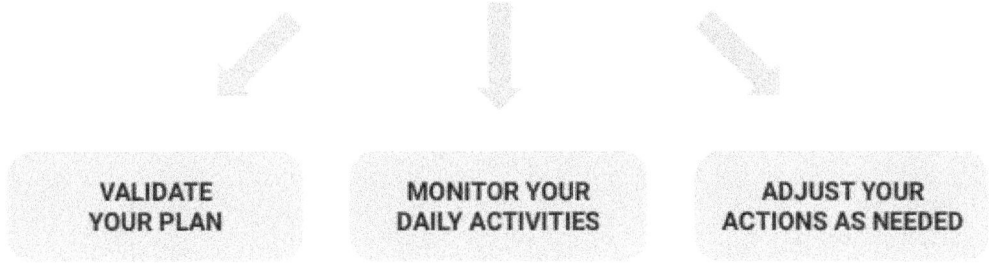

In Phase One and the first two chapters of Phase Two, we explored gaining clarity about where you are and where you want to go. This was followed by practical aspects of creating a sugar-free lifestyle and action steps to help you get there. In this chapter, you will learn the benefits of self-monitoring and techniques that you can use to identify problems before you go wildly off track and instead adjust as needed.

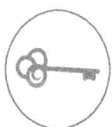

Key Concepts

The Benefits of Keeping a Daily Journal

Journaling is a powerful tool that you can use to brainstorm, track your progress, and help you keep moving forward with clarity. Writing provides insight that allows you to better connect with your intention and enables you to process the changes you are making. It also helps you identify where you are struggling and think about what you might do differently. It is not just about documenting what you are eating, but journaling other aspects of your experience can be a source of clarity that provides direction and information you can use to push yourself forward in a way that aligns with your unique needs.

The benefits of keeping a daily sugar-free lifestyle journal to track your progress include:

- **Accountability**. Recording what you eat or what activities you do every day provides a daily reality check. For many people, the knowledge that they will have to record their results provides extra motivation to stay on track.
- **Removing Roadblocks**. If you are vigilant about using the journal, you will see patterns of behavior emerge and be able to identify patterns holding you back. The more "health" data you have, the better you'll be able to adjust your patterns and fix problem spots easily.
- **Motivation**. Seeing your progress in black and white helps you to carry on when your motivation is fading. If you find yourself floundering or far afield from your goals, one of the best ways to get back on track is to use your daily journal.
- **Facilitating Troubleshooting**. If you do not achieve your expected results, recording your activities will make it much easier to work with health providers to evaluate what you have been doing and identify where you might adjust to reach your goals.

Daily Journal Tools and Techniques

There are several different ways to monitor your progress. In today's world, one popular approach is to use online applications to track your daily food and exercise. Although these applications can be beneficial, in the beginning, I strongly recommend using a daily journal to monitor your progress, build motivation, and refine your action plan as needed.

Methods available to keep a daily journal include:

- Published journals with templates to track food consumption and daily activities,
- Blank journals where you can choose which information to track, and

- Online notetaking applications are available where you can enter information in an electronic tool and have the benefits of electronic storage and convenience.

Choose a method that works best for you. The important thing is to use a format that enables you to track information consistently to:

- Reinforce successful habits so that they become a natural part of your daily routine,
- Raise your awareness about what you eat daily, and
- Monitor your activities so that you can adjust your actions as needed.

As you begin to assimilate success habits into your daily routine, you may find that you don't need to use a journal every day. But you can always come back to it during times of stress or periods where you need extra help to stay on track.

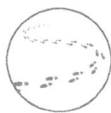

Action Steps

Track Your Daily Food Consumption and Other Activities

You can record your food consumption and related daily activities in a blank journal, print and use the journal template provided, download the journal sheets supplied in the Sugar-Free Lifestyle Community, or purchase a different journal that meets your needs.

What to Track in Your Daily Journal

For optimum results, you should track enough information to see patterns of behavior emerge. This will enable you to gain a better understanding of how to develop and maintain successful habits that support your ability to maintain your sugar-free lifestyle. Here is a list of items to track:

- Each day, track the food you are consuming.

- Note when you consume your food (Breakfast, Lunch, Dinner, Snack). If you are also testing your blood sugar levels, this will enable you to correlate food consumption with any blood glucose results that are higher than desired.
- If you are diabetic, monitor your blood glucose levels, noting the result and time of testing.
- Each day, incorporate an activity to reduce your stress level.
- Keep track of the amount of water or tea consumed.
- Note the amount of time you spend exercising. (Walking, jogging, aerobics, etc.)

Some people also like to maintain a daily gratitude entry in their journal, along with notes that provide insight into challenges they faced and accomplishments that encourage them to keep moving forward. For example, if you found yourself consuming added sugar, you might write down what you ate, when you consumed the food, how you felt at the time, and what you might do differently when cravings for this food arise.

FOOD TRACKER
DATE:

BREAKFAST
TIME:

_____
_____
_____
_____

50% NON-STARCHY VEGETABLES
25% HIGH QUALITY PROTEIN
25% OTHER*

LUNCH
TIME:

_____
_____
_____
_____

Cross out 1 bottle for each Serving of Water Consumed
1 bottle = 8 ounces

DINNER
TIME:

_____
_____
_____
_____

Blood Sugar Testing Results:

Time:
Result:

SNACKS
TIME(S):

_____
_____
_____

Time:
Result:

Time:
Result:

TODAY, I AM GRATEFUL FOR:

"Stress Busters"
1 heart = 15 minutes

Exercise
1 figure = 1/2 hr

Maintain a Weekly "Crowd out" Tracker (Optional)

Since the Sugar-Free Lifestyle Food Plan strategy involves crowding out sugar from various sources and adding in foods for daily consumption, you may also want to keep track of the foods you crowd out daily.

- The goal is to Crowd Out foods that cause fast/sharp rises in blood sugar and insulin.
- In the Added Sugar and "Hidden Sugar" Sections, for each day in the week, place a checkmark in the column associated with the food and day that you did not consume that food.
- In the Fruit, Dairy, Natural Sugar section, place a checkmark in the column associated with the food and day that describes your consumption of that item. (For example, if you sparingly consumed low/ medium glycemic food, put a check next to that item. If you ate several servings of low/ medium glycemic fruit, leave the box blank.)

DATE:

	SUN	MON	TUE	WED	THU	FRI	SAT
ADDED SUGAR							
No beverages with added sugar							
No soda with added sugar							
(No diet soda)							
No recipes with added sugar							
No salad dressings with added sugar							
No processed foods with added sugar							
No yogurt with added sugar							
No high fructose corn syrup							
No yogurt with added sugar							
HIDDEN SUGAR							
No Grain-Based flour bread							
No Grain-Based flour crackers, muffins, tortillas, cookies, cakes, snacks							
No white potatoes							

	SUN	MON	TUE	WED	THU	FRI	SAT
No wheat-based pasta (small amounts of high protein wheat mixed with lupini bean flour, or other types of wheat pasta alternatives OK)							
NO or very small portion of whole grains (Small amount of steel-cut oats, barley, quinoa OK)							
FRUIT, DAIRY, NATURAL SUGAR							
No high glycemic fruit (a small piece of non-ripe banana is OK in a smoothie)							
If desired, consume medium/low glycemic fruit sparingly.							
If desired, consume lactose dairy or lactose free dairy products in moderation.							

Takeaways & Highlights

In this chapter, you learned the benefits of self-monitoring and techniques that you can use to identify problems before you go wildly off track and instead adjust as needed.

The benefits of keeping a daily sugar-free lifestyle journal to track your progress include:

- Accountability
- Removing Roadblocks
- Motivation
- Facilitating Troubleshooting

Methods available to keep a daily journal include:

- Published journals with templates to track food consumption and daily activities

- Blank journals where you can choose which information to track
- Online notetaking applications are available where you can enter information in an electronic tool and have the benefits of electronic storage and convenience.

List of items to track in your daily journal:

- Each day, track the food you are consuming.
- Note when you consume your food (Breakfast, Lunch, Dinner, Snack). If you are also testing your blood sugar levels, this will enable you to correlate the consumption of foods with any blood glucose results that are higher than desired.
- If you are diabetic, monitor your blood glucose levels, noting the result and time of testing.
- Each day, incorporate an activity to reduce your stress level.
- Keep track of the amount of water or tea consumed.
- Note the amount of time you spend exercising. (Walking, jogging, aerobics, etc.)
- Optional: Gratitude Entries, Notes/Observations

Since the Sugar-Free Lifestyle Food Plan strategy involves crowding out sugar from various sources and adding In foods for daily consumption, you may also want to keep track of the foods you crowd out daily.

CHAPTER 14
Enhance Your Food Plan with Exercise, Restful Sleep, and Stress Management

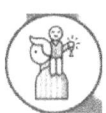

Coach on Your Shoulder

The Three Pillars of Vibrant Health

Ultimately, the path to thriving with a sugar-free lifestyle is about creating a balanced life based on three pillars of vibrant health, as shown in the diagram below.

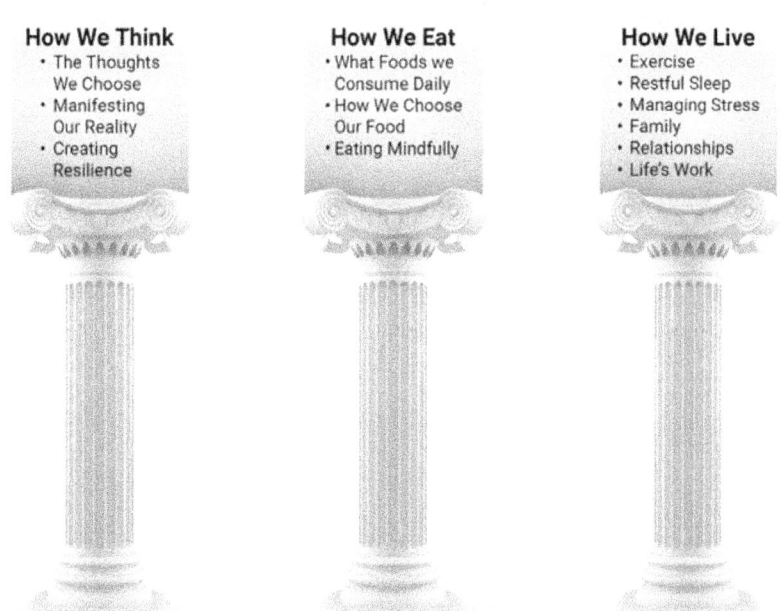

The World Health Organization (WHO) defines health as a state of complete physical, mental, social, and spiritual well-being, and not merely an absence of disease or infirmity. With this in mind, each step in the Sugar-Free Lifestyle Roadmap™ has been designed to lead you toward your vision of health at all levels: physically, mentally, and spiritually.

As we have discovered in the previous chapters, eliminating foods that cause roller-coaster blood sugars is a foundation of physical wellness, along with embracing change and creating resilience. Both how you think and how you eat are two essential aspects of living a sugar-free lifestyle. The third and equally important component is how you live, including moving your body on a regular basis, getting restful sleep, and managing stress. All of these affect your ability to stay on track with a sugar-free lifestyle and keep blood sugars under control. In this chapter, we will focus on the third pillar, How We Live.

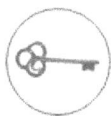

Key Concepts

Exercise Benefits, Tips, and Guidelines

Exercise is a potent tool in your journey to a sugar-free lifestyle. By incorporating exercise into your daily routine, you'll experience a range of benefits, including clearing the blood of glucose, boosting insulin sensitivity, improving heart and cardiovascular health, and aiding your body in fat burning.

- Regular exercise helps your cells become more sensitive to insulin. When this happens, your insulin is more effective, and your cells use more glucose. This sensitivity to insulin and the benefit of lower blood glucose levels last for several hours, even after the activity has ended.
- In addition to glucose entering your bloodstream from the food you eat, your liver also produces glucose from stored glycogen. This is a normal function of the liver, but sometimes it makes more glucose than your body can use, causing your blood glucose level to go up. Regular activity can help counter this effect.

- Building muscle mass not only makes you stronger but also helps your body burn fat through an efficient process called thermogenesis. This process creates heat for your body by burning excess calories from your fat supplies. It starts by mobilizing fat from fat cells, transporting it through the blood to muscle cells, where it's converted into soluble fat and burned for energy. The more muscle you have, the more fat you can burn for energy.

Getting Into the Fat Burning Zone

First, you need to have a basic understanding of muscle fiber. There are three types of fibers present in voluntary muscles. (Voluntary muscle tissue is the skeletal muscle that moves your body when stimulated by your intention or reaction).

Fast Twitch. This muscle type is responsible for explosive movements. When you're lifting heavy weights or sprinting, it's these fibers that kick into action. Their primary source of energy is the blood sugar stored in the muscle cells, as well as in the blood and the liver. Unlike other muscle types, fast twitch fibers don't rely on fat for fuel, but on the quick energy provided by sugars.

Medium/Middle Twitch. This muscle tissue also responds to a demand for explosive, high-intensity activity. (such as boxing, playing basketball, or intensive aerobics) Middle twitch fiber is capable of longer periods of activity and does not have the strength capacity of the fast twitch fiber. Like fast twitch fiber, middle twitch is also fueled by readily available sugars, not fat.

Slow twitch. These muscle fibers utilize fat as a source of fuel. Exercise that requires a long period of consistent activity is the type of exercise that relies on the slow twitch fibers. For example, cyclists and long-distance runners primarily use their body fat as fuel, burning it during a process known as the Krebs cycle. Through this cycle, the body metabolizes fat into energy. The Krebs cycle occurs when you have done at least 5 minutes of rhythmic low intensity activity, creating a slow but steady demand for more energy. The body will then call on its fat stores and turns the fat into energy.

What are some of the best exercises to help you burn fat? Paced walking, slow jogging, or any exercise that enables you to keep your heart rate in the fat burning zone.

How do you know when you are in the fat burning zone? First, you need to find your target heart rate to find your fat burning zone (subtract your age from 220). If your age is 45, subtract 45 from

220. 220-45=175, meaning that 175 heartbeats per minute is your maximum heart rate. To burn fat effectively, your goal is to keep your heart rate between 55%-65% of your maximum heart rate. Ideally, the closer you are to 65%, the better. If you are extremely out of shape, you should start at 50% of your maximum and work up to 65%.

Types of Exercise to Consider

When thinking about what types of activities to include, you can break exercise into several categories:

- Physical Activity, which is any movement that uses energy, such as climbing the stairs, mowing the lawn, or walking an extra row in the parking lot to get to your car.
- Aerobic Exercise that can be thought of as more vigorous, continuous, and concerted movement like dancing, walking, running, rebounding, or bicycling.
- Recreational Activities such as golf, bowling, tennis, and hiking.
- Flexibility and Strength Activities, which are very beneficial for relieving emotional tension and stress. Examples of these activities include stretching, yoga, tai chi, and strength training. Strength training is also important for building muscle mass.

Ideally, your overall plan should include all four exercise categories. But, if you are not already active, just getting started with some extra physical activity will be beneficial. Exactly how often you should and can exercise depends on many factors, including your:

- Overall health,
- Blood glucose levels and control,

- Lifestyle,
- Fitness goals, and
- Diabetes complications, if relevant.

The key is to incorporate exercise into your daily routine in a way that aligns with your lifestyle and health goals.

Exercise: Tips to Get Moving

- **Find out how active you are**. Investing in a tool to monitor your physical activity is a great way to determine where you stand. Monitoring physical activity can enhance personal health and fitness by providing tangible data on various types of movement, such as steps taken throughout the day. If you are sedentary, setting goals for daily steps, often recommended at 10,000 steps, can help you get started with more physical activity, which is linked to improved cardiovascular health, better weight management, and enhanced mood. If you take less than 10,000 steps daily, you can set goals for getting more steps into your day by averaging your step counts for three days and determining how many steps you would need to average 10,000 steps per day.
- **If desired, use a device to track physical activities**. There are many different types to choose from, including pedometers and wearable activity monitors. A pedometer is a simple device that counts the number of steps a person takes by detecting motion with each step. More advanced wearable devices, such as fitness trackers and smartwatches, not only track steps but also monitor other aspects of physical activity like distance traveled, calories burned, and even heart rate. By offering real-time feedback, these tools can help you stay motivated, adjust your activity levels as needed, and achieve your fitness goals.
- **Identify some exercise activities you would like to try**. Consider what would fit into your daily routine. Some people enjoy going to the gym. Others would much prefer to take a walk in the park or participate in online classes in the privacy of their living room. Write down some activities you think you would actually do, and visualize when and how often you would do that activity in a

week. Set goals that work for you. Plan to begin gradually and increase the intensity and duration of your workouts over time.
- **Make a schedule**. It's easy to allow busy schedules and other activities to interfere with an activity plan. To avoid breaking your momentum, develop an exercise schedule and make it a priority. Consider what time of the day and which days of the week are best for your activity. Think of your exercise time as a date you make with yourself, one that you wouldn't break or ignore any more than you would consciously miss an appointment with someone else. If you find it helpful, write your activity schedule in a calendar or daily planner.
- **Be flexible**. Having said how important it is to make a schedule, it is also important not to make yourself crazy over exercising. If you do, you may grow to resent it and find yourself avoiding it altogether. The important thing is to keep moving on a regular basis. If you miss a day or two, the best thing you can do is to engage in some form of activity to get back into your routine, and don't beat yourself up for taking a few days off from exercising.
- **Find a buddy**. Activities and exercise are often more fun when you do them with someone else. Also, a partner can help you stay motivated and give you someone to compare your progress with.
- Build in Variety: The worst thing that you can do is become so bored with your exercise routine that you don't want to do it. The best way to avoid this is to find several different types of activities that you enjoy and do them on different days of the week. You can even make your time in front of the TV count by working out on an exercise bike or treadmill while you watch your favorite show.
- **Try rebounding**. Rebounding applies weight and movement to every cell, causing the entire body to become stronger and more flexible. It's fun, and rebounding is great for diabetics because it increases circulation, strengthens the heart, muscles and bones, and improves cell efficiency. Check with your doctor to make sure it is a form of exercise that is OK for you, and make sure you invest in a high-quality rebound unit that is designed properly so that you won't sustain injuries to your knees, ankles, or joints.
- **Make exercise fun**. There will be days when doing any exercise feels like too much effort. The trick is to figure out ways to make your exercise as much fun

as possible so that you will want to do it when you aren't feeling motivated. Dancing is one of the more fun ways to exercise. Today, many innovative dance fitness classes are available in person and online, and the best part is once you learn the routines, you can put on some music and do them anytime. Think of your exercise as a gift that you give to yourself. Who wouldn't want a present that helps you stay in shape and feel great at the same time?

Exercise: Safety Guidelines

- **If you are under a doctor's care for any physical condition, clear any exercise program with your physician before getting started**. This is essential for diabetics. In addition to assessing your overall physical health, your doctor can determine the kinds of exercise that are right for you. This decision will take into account certain types of exercise you should avoid if you have diabetic complications such as retinopathy, heart disease, or nerve damage.
- **Start any new exercise routine slowly, with a gradual buildup**. For example, if you are starting a walking program, begin with just 10 minutes a day and gradually work up to 30 or 60 minutes a day.
- **Stop whenever you don't feel well**. If you feel pain or pressure in any area of your body during the exercise activity or experience shakiness, dizziness, faintness, blurry vision, or headaches, discontinue the activity and inform your physician.
- **Be consistent**. If you make some form of exercise part of your daily routine, you will get better results and avoid injury.
- **Drink plenty of fluids**. This is important for anyone participating in an exercise session, whether or not they have diabetes. Drink before, during, and after exercise if your session lasts over 20 minutes.
- **Make attentive foot care an integral part of your exercise program**. Peripheral nerve damage can lead to a loss of sensation in the feet, which means a blister can go unnoticed and become infected. To avoid problems with your feet, buy fitness shoes that fit well, break them in slowly, and wear clean socks every time you exercise. After exercising, check your feet for blisters, redness, or tenderness, and talk with your healthcare team if you experience any of these problems.

Why Restful Sleep Matters

Sleep deprivation raises levels of ghrelin, the hunger hormone, and decreases levels of leptin, the hormone that makes us feel full. To compensate for lower energy levels, people who sleep poorly may seek out high carbohydrate foods that drain their energy and cause roller-coaster blood sugar levels. The good news is that when you get enough sleep, you will have more energy, less stress, and a better mindset for choosing foods that support your health.

Roller coaster blood sugar levels and sleep are intricately connected, and many people with high blood sugar experience issues with getting a good night's sleep. Both high blood sugar (hyperglycemia) and low blood sugar (hypoglycemia) during the night can affect sleep in several ways, including the inability to fall asleep (insomnia), restless sleep, and interrupted sleep --- all can also lead to fatigue and other related problems. If you find yourself waking up to use the bathroom, it could be that you drank too much liquid too close to bedtime, or when blood sugar levels are high, the kidneys overcompensate by causing you to urinate more often. During the night, these frequent trips to the bathroom lead to disrupted sleep.

In addition to the immediate frustration of sleepless nights, lack of good sleep can cause problems the next day. Sleep deprivation raises levels of ghrelin, the hunger hormone, and decreases levels of leptin, the hormone that makes us feel full. To compensate for lower energy levels, people who sleep poorly may be more likely to seek relief in foods that raise blood sugar and put them at risk of chronic high blood sugar levels or obesity, both of which are risk factors for diabetes. People who experience disturbed sleep or frequent nighttime awakenings may also be less likely to stick with their diabetes self-care routines, including eating foods that support blood sugar control, getting enough exercise, and closely monitoring blood glucose levels.

Even if you are not diabetic or pre-diabetic, sleep deprivation raises the risk of developing insulin resistance. The good news is that you can change your habits, including eliminating foods that cause roller coaster blood sugar levels, staying active, and creating a nighttime routine to improve sleep quality. When you get enough sleep, you'll be more alert, have more energy, experience less stress, and have a better mindset for managing your food throughout the day.

Tips for Getting Enough Quality Rest

- **Focus on controlling your blood sugar levels during the day and early evening**. Managing blood sugar levels is your first defense against a restless night. When your blood sugar levels are too high or too low, this can wake you up at night. One of the best things for better sleep is eliminating roller-coaster blood sugar levels by adhering to a quality carbohydrate diet plan that avoids foods that cause a sharp rise in blood sugar levels followed by a flood of insulin and blood sugar crashes. If you are diabetic and you want to see if your blood sugar is spiking or going too low in the middle of the night, try checking it around 2 or 3 o'clock to see if you are having an issue. If you find that high or low blood sugar levels are interfering with your sleep, you can talk to your doctor about possible causes and what to do.
- **Don't eat a heavy meal in the evening before bedtime.** Nighttime eating is a common issue for many people. It is generally a good idea to avoid eating food close to bedtime. If you want a light snack, it should be eaten 1-2 hours before bedtime and include a combo of protein and quality carbohydrates that do not spike blood sugar levels.
- **Moderate consumption of caffeine and alcohol**. Alcohol and liquids containing caffeine, such as black tea, coffee, soda, and hot chocolate interfere with your ability to fall asleep and overall sleep quality. For a better night's sleep, avoid drinking alcoholic beverages later in the evening, and limit the amount of caffeine you consume throughout the day with the goal of eliminating it several hours before bed. Although having a piece of chocolate before bed might seem comforting, avoid this. Chocolate has caffeine, and caffeine can keep you awake. As long as it is not a personal trigger food, a small piece of sugar-free dark chocolate is OK. Just have it earlier in the day.
- **Limit the consumption of liquids 1-2 hours before going to sleep**. If you find it relaxing to drink an herbal tea such as chamomile or a drink that contains magnesium, try not to drink tea or other liquids close to bedtime to avoid

waking up in the middle of the night for a bathroom break. Make it a habit to use the bathroom right before you go to bed.

- **Set and maintain a consistent bedtime**. Going to bed and waking up at the same time each night helps regulate your body's internal clock. It helps your body know when to release calming hormones to fall asleep and stimulate hormones to wake up naturally. If possible, make a plan to go to bed at the same time every day, even on the weekends. By establishing a consistent bedtime, you enhance the quality of your sleep, which supports better stress management and reduces the likelihood of turning to sugar for energy or comfort. If you enjoy taking naps, keep them relatively short—around 20 to 30 minutes—and limit them to the early afternoon. Napping any later is likely to interfere with your ability to get to sleep at night
- **Fall asleep in your bedroom, not on the sofa**. Another common issue for many is falling asleep on the sofa and then going to bed. This can interrupt your sleep pattern, making it difficult to get back to sleep once you get into bed. Create a bedroom oasis and go into your bedroom before falling asleep.
- **Develop a bedtime ritual that includes relaxing activities**. Finding ways to relax before bed is important to counteract the effects of daily stress. Finish exercise, chores, and errands at least an hour before you go to bed. Then, wind down and relax one to two hours before bed to help your body get ready for sleep. Consider a gentle yoga routine, breathing exercises, reading, listening to calm music, writing in a journal, or a warm bath.
- **Create a peaceful, sleep-friendly environment**. When it comes to getting a good night's rest, the environment in your bedroom makes a significant difference. Ever wonder why you sleep so well in a comfy hotel room? It is mainly because good hotels focus on creating a relaxing environment. Start by taking a look around your bedroom. Is it cluttered, full of electronic equipment or other distractions? Keeping your bedroom uncluttered, a comfortable temperature, dark at night, and quiet while you sleep can significantly improve your sleep. Television, smartphones, tablets, and even clock radios that are too bright can interfere with your ability to fall and stay asleep. I am not against having TVs or tablets for reading in the bedroom, as long as they are turned off

at least 30 minutes before you fall asleep. If you need to have your cell phone by your bed, change the settings to only receive messages that are emergencies

- **If you currently use your bedroom as an office, rethink this arrangement**. Make your bedroom a place to rest, not get distracted or reminded of stressful situations. I originally had my office in my bedroom and realized that it was causing underlying anxiety, so I moved it to a corner of my dining room instead. If you live in a small space, and this is impossible, consider a piece of furniture designed to let you keep your office out of view in the evening.

When Should You See Your Doctor for Ongoing Concerns?

If you have concerns or adopting basic lifestyle changes doesn't improve your sleep, it's important to talk to your doctor. Conditions that affect sleep can be serious and may lead to long-term health issues over time. Your doctor can assess whether you have a more significant sleep issue, such as diabetic neuropathy, nighttime eating syndrome, or sleep apnea, and recommend further tests or treatment.

Managing Stress

Stress is a normal and natural response to challenges in life. Stressful events trigger a series of chemical reactions in your body, including producing hormones such as cortisol and adrenalin that are designed to protect you.

Experiencing stress is not necessarily a bad thing, and your body is designed to handle a certain amount of stress. In the "old days," the reaction was designed to enable humans to protect themselves from threats and starvation. One of the jobs of cortisol is to quickly break down available sugars, fats, and proteins to supply energy. So the caveman had the energy needed to get away from the dinosaur!!!

In a more modern example, if you step off a curb and a car comes speeding towards you, your body responds to help you react. At the outset of this event, your body will have a physical reaction, such as shallow breathing or a feeling that your heart is racing. This triggers the release of two hormones: adrenalin and cortisol. In a stressful situation, cortisol quickly breaks down available sugars, fats and proteins to supply energy so that you can get out of the way of the car coming towards you. Then, once the "crisis" is over, your body returns to normal.

The Damaging Effects of Chronic Stress

When stress becomes chronic or unmanaged, the constant release of stress hormones begins to have negative effects, including increased hunger, cravings, and high blood sugar levels. If you are an emotional eater and try to reduce stressful feelings with food, especially sugar, chronic stress results in a vicious cycle of eating and feeling out of control with no end in sight

Unfortunately, in today's world, we experience "Chronic Stress" from all directions, including finances, career, deadlines, lack of time, family, the environment, and world events. Your body can't tell the difference between stress from a car speeding towards you and the stress you feel when bills are late. Even dieting can be perceived by your body as a source of stress because another job of cortisol is to protect your fat stores so that they are available when food is unavailable. If you subject yourself to artificial famine, your body considers itself to be under stress, and cortisol is released in response.

When cortisol is released, it tries to supply energy to deal with the stressful situation. But if you constantly feel stressed out and no ready energy source is available, cortisol begins to steal nitrogen from the structural protein in your muscles. It converts the protein to sugar for energy, and the end result is the ongoing destruction of the muscle tissue needed to burn fat. When stress is constant and continues unmanaged, this process repeats itself over and over again.

Ongoing stress also increases carbohydrate cravings and decreases serotonin levels, causing you to crave sweets and carbohydrates. Over time, the effects of chronic stress and high levels of cortisol take a toll on both your mental and physical state, and it is critical to take some time out for self-care to reduce chronic stress by practicing stress-relieving activities such as meditation, deep breathing, or spending time in nature.

Additionally, losing muscle mass is a significant problem if you are trying to lose weight because fat is burned within your muscle cells for energy. The more muscle you carry, the more fat you can burn for energy, and studies show that losing even 1 ounce of muscle mass lowers the body's ability to create energy and reduces your fat burning ability.

Bottom Line: The combination of being in a constant state of stress plus consuming foods that cause intense glucose spikes results in more fat storage with a decreased ability to lose it as high cortisol levels diminish your ability to burn fat!

De-stressing is not a luxury; it is necessary for your health and maintaining a sugar-free lifestyle. The tips below are designed to help you address the underlying chronic stress that often fuels the consumption of sugar and other trigger foods.

Tips for Managing Chronic Stress in Your Daily Life

- **Include Daily De-Stressing Activities**. Incorporating de-stressing activities into your daily routine helps manage stress levels, reducing the need to rely on sugar as a coping mechanism. Regularly engaging in these activities builds resilience against stress and weakens the association between stress and sugar consumption
- **Practice Deep Breathing**. When you are stressed or anxious, your breathing tends to be irregular and shallow. Deep breathing activates the relaxation response in your body by accessing the lower portion of your lungs. Calming your nervous system can be helpful both for day-to-day anxiety as well as ongoing generalized anxiety disorder
- **Prioritize Your Health and Take Time for Yourself**. Prioritizing your health sends a powerful message to yourself that your well-being is important. When you consistently take time for yourself, you're more likely to manage stress in ways that don't involve turning to sugar, helping you change your relationship with it over time
- **Exercise Regularly**. Exercise is a natural stress reliever, releasing endorphins that improve mood and reduce anxiety. Regular physical activity not only helps regulate blood sugar levels but helps to manage high blood sugar levels, lower stress, and reduce sugar cravings.
- **Write in a Journal.** Journaling is an effective way to process stressful situations. It allows you to identify your feelings, gain clarity about the sources

of stress in your life, and develop strategies to cope with stress in healthier ways, rather than resorting to sugar or other trigger foods.
- **Practice Gratitude & Enjoy Life**. Practicing gratitude shifts your focus away from stress and toward positive aspects of your life. Finding joy in non-food-related activities and appreciating life's simple pleasures helps you shift your attention away from negative emotions, calm anxiety, and keep your thoughts focused on the present.
- **Develop a Support System**. Trying to manage stressful situations on your own can lead to frustration and hopelessness, leading to a vicious cycle of chronic stress. Reaching out for help from a peer group, friend, family member, physician, health coach, or therapist provides another perspective that can shed light on possible solutions and help you take action to relieve the feelings of distress and anxiety that you are experiencing. This, in turn, empowers you to take action and rely less on sugar and other trigger foods as a coping mechanism.
- **Eliminate added sugar and other trigger foods**. Avoiding foods that cause a sharp rise in blood glucose levels and intense insulin response will decrease the constant pattern of sugar highs and subsequent crashes that lead to feelings of anxiety, exhaustion, and overwhelm.

Managing Chronic Stress: Deep Breathing Exercise

When you are stressed or experiencing anxiety, your breathing tends to be shallow. This is known as chest breathing, and it occurs without your diaphragm assisting the breathing process.

Focused diaphragmatic breathing, sometimes known as belly breathing, involves breathing slowly and using the diaphragm to open up your lungs and breathe more efficiently. This type of breathing signals your nervous system to calm your body down, and practicing deep breathing will help you feel calm and energized even after you have completed your deep breathing exercise.

Take a moment to practice deep breathing when you are feeling stressed or anxious, and if possible, repeat this exercise a few times throughout the day. This is also a great way to relax as part of your evening sleep routine.

Here is the basic technique:

- Sit in a tall chair with your back straight and shoulders relaxed, or lie down on a comfortable flat surface with your knees bent and feet flat.
- Gently place one hand on your stomach and the other on your chest.
- Breathe in slowly through your nose, filling your lungs until you can't take in any more air.
- As you breathe in, feel the air moving through your nostrils down into your abdomen, expanding your stomach while your chest remains relatively still. The hand on your chest should remain still, while the one on your belly should rise.
- Hold for 3 seconds.
- Then slightly purse your lips (as if sipping through a straw) and exhale slowly through your lips until all of the air is gone, and feel your stomach contracting as you exhale.
- Repeat these breathing steps 2-5 times in one session.

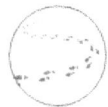

Action Steps

Primary Food Assessment: Movement and Exercise

In the chart below, place a checkmark in the column associated with your level of agreement with each corresponding statement.

How often do you agree with each statement below?	Never	Sometimes	Often	Daily
I engage in some form of physical activity such as walking, climbing stairs, yard work, housework, or moving around at work.				
I participate in aerobic activities such as dance fitness classes, swimming, running, or aerobic-paced walking.				

I lift weights or engage in other strength training activities.				
I play sports such as tennis, basketball, soccer, baseball, or pickleball.				
I track my fitness level, such as time spent exercising each day or steps taken daily.				
I enjoy being physically active.				
I am able to move freely with little or no pain or restriction.				

On a scale of 1-10 (10 being the highest level/High Priority and 1 being the lowest level/Low Priority) what is your priority level for being physically active in order to reach your life and health goals?

Based on your answers to the Assessment above, what are the top three issues that affect your ability to become more active? (Examples: *I don't enjoy exercise, I rarely engage in aerobic or strength training, and I tend to be very sedentary*).

Based on your existing movement challenges, what is your immediate #1 goal? (Example: *to engage in a form of aerobic activity for 1 hour 3 times a week*).

What are two other goals that you would like to achieve in the next six months to a year?

What types of activities could you realistically incorporate into your routine over the next month to achieve the goal you identified as your top priority? (Examples: *Leave work early, schedule exercise into my calendar, walk for an hour at least 2 times a week, join a dance fitness class, watch less TV*).

What are the biggest obstacles you face moving more and establishing an exercise routine? (Example: *very busy work schedule, including working late hours, too tired to work out*).

What could you do to overcome those obstacles? (Examples: *manage my work schedule to allow time for exercise and get enough sleep at night*).

Do you need help getting started or staying consistent? If yes, what steps will you commit to in order to get the support you need?

What would the benefits be if you were moving/exercising more regularly? (Examples: *more energy, better mood, managed blood sugar levels and weight, less desire to eat sweets*).

What are the "costs" of not engaging in enough physical activity? (Examples: *poor health, inability to participate in activities because of lack of stamina*).

List 2-4 specific action steps that you will take to either get started with including physical activity into your daily/weekly routine or to become more consistent. (Examples: *leave work at 5:00 three days a week and walk for an hour in the park near my home, bring my exercise clothes to work and change into them before leaving, find and enroll in a dance fitness class*). **When you are ready, implement your Action Steps.**

Primary Food Assessment: Restful Sleep

In the chart below, place a checkmark in the column associated with your level of agreement with each corresponding statement.

How often do you agree with each statement below?	Never	Sometimes	Often	Daily
I get 7-8 hours of restful sleep.				
I wake up during the night to use the bathroom.				
I wake up during the night feeling hungry and engage in nighttime eating.				
I wake up in the morning feeling refreshed and energized.				
It is hard for me to fall asleep.				
I follow a routine to relax and get ready for sleep.				

How often do you agree with each statement below?	Never	Sometimes	Often	Daily
I have a consistent bedtime.				
I go to sleep before midnight.				
I stop eating at least 2 hours before bedtime.				
I fall asleep at night in a chair or sofa.				
I keep my bedroom clutter-free and comfortable for a relaxing night's sleep.				
I get tired during the day.				
I take naps.				
I stop consuming caffeine at least 2 hours before bedtime.				

On a scale of 1-10 (10 being the highest level/High Priority and 1 being the lowest level/Low Priority) what is your priority level for taking action to experience sufficient, restful sleep?

Based on your answers to the Assessment above, what are the top three issues that keep you from getting enough quality sleep? (Examples: *I fall asleep on the sofa watching TV, I consume too many liquids close to bedtime, and my bedroom is very chaotic*).

Based on your existing sleep challenges, what is your immediate #1 goal? (Example: *To establish a regular routine and go upstairs to bed by 11:00 pm*).

What are two other goals that you would like to achieve in the next six months to a year?

What types of activities could you realistically incorporate into your routine over the next month to achieve the goal you identified as your top priority? (Examples: *Turn off the television, take my evening medications at a specified time, stop falling asleep on the sofa*).

What challenges could prevent you from engaging in these activities or establishing habits that support more restful sleep?? (Example: *eating foods at night that spike my blood sugars, making me feel too exhausted to comply with my routine*).

What could you do to overcome those obstacles? (Examples: *eat a balanced sugar-free dinner and stop snacking in the evening*).

Do you need help getting started or staying consistent? If yes, what steps will you commit to in order to get the support you need?

What would the benefits be to you if you were getting better quality sleep? (Examples: *more energy, better mood, managed blood sugar levels and weight, less desire to eat sweets*).

What are the "costs" to you if you don't get sufficient quality sleep? (Examples: *poor health, inability to participate in activities because of lack of stamina*).

List 2-4 specific action steps that you will take to support more restful sleep. (Examples: *stop eating snacks at night, take my medications at a consistent time each evening, go upstairs to my bedroom by 11:00*).**When you are ready, implement your Action Steps.**

Primary Food Assessment: Managing Chronic Stress

How often do you agree with each statement below?	Never	Sometimes	Often	Daily
I experience anxiety that affects my ability to function.				
I spend at least 30 minutes engaging in a de-stressing activity, such as yoga, meditation, or a massage.				
I spend 5-10 minutes practicing deep breathing exercises.				

I write in a journal to explore and express my thoughts, feelings, and experiences.				
I engage in physical activity for at least 30 minutes.				
I set aside dedicated time for self-care and to relax and have fun.				
I consume caffeine to maintain alertness.				
I eat sugar and other trigger foods in reaction to stressful situations.				
I have insomnia when I am stressed or worried.				
I find myself worrying over things I cannot control.				
I procrastinate and find it difficult to complete tasks when I am feeling stressed.				
I reach out for help when I encounter situations that cause stress in my life.				
When stressed, I take time to gain perspective and consider how this stressful situation fits into my bigger life picture.				
I practice gratitude in various ways (such as writing in a gratitude journal, letting others know that I appreciate them, and acknowledging things that I am grateful for).				
My energy level is high, and I look forward to my day.				
I feel exhausted and want to sleep or zone out.				
I experience physical symptoms of stress (such as heart palpitations, racing heart, tightness in my chest, stomach upset, skin issues, and hair falling out).				

Many situations can cause us stress. Place an "X" in the column on the right next to those you've experienced in the last six months.

The death of your partner, family member, or friend.	
Death of a pet.	
Getting ready to move or have recently moved to a new home.	
Let go from employment, or looking for a new job.	
Changed jobs or recently started a new career.	
Long work hours (10+ hours/day).	
Ongoing pressure and demands at work or school.	
Recently retired.	
Debt or other financial pressures.	
Significant or frequent travel.	
Fast-paced/busy/rushed life.	
New Relationship.	
New Marriage.	
Ongoing relationship problems with partner(s).	
Relationship breakup/divorce or separation.	
Ongoing problems with other family, relatives, or friends.	
Pregnancy /new baby.	
Caring for child(ren).	
Caring for a sick, disabled, and/or older family member or friend.	
A child left home.	
Other changes to family situation (such as an aging parent moving in).	
Major physical health problem (either acute or chronic).	
Substance abuse issues and/or another addiction.	
Heavy athletic training or athletic competition.	
Other:	

On a scale of 1-10 (10 being the highest level/extreme stress and 1 being the lowest level/no stress), what is your stress level on a typical day? (within the last two weeks)

On a scale of 1-10 (10 being the highest level/my life is panicked and feels out of control, and 1 being the lowest level/my life is calm and relaxed), where are you in terms of managing your life and schedule most of the time?

On a scale of 1-10 (10 being the highest level/High Priority and 1 being the lowest level/Low Priority), what is your priority level for taking action to manage chronic stress in your life?

Based on your answers to the Assessment on the previous pages, what are the top 3 issues that you want to address to manage chronic stress? (Examples: *Not taking time to relax, worrying about things I cannot control, overscheduling my time*).

Based on your existing stress levels and challenges managing stress, what is your immediate #1 goal? (Examples: *Taking ½ hour each day to incorporate a "stress-buster" into my routine*).

What types of activities could you realistically incorporate into your routine over the next month to achieve the goal you identified as a top priority? (Example: *Meditation sessions before bedtime, writing in my journal*, seeking assistance for my anxiety).

What are your biggest obstacles to managing chronic stress on a daily basis? (Examples: *turning to food instead of more helpful activities, inconsistency, constant worrying*).

What could you do to overcome those obstacles? (Examples: *slow down, get and use a "worry box," seek assistance*).

Do you need help getting started or staying consistent? If yes, what steps will you commit to in order to get the support you need?

What would the benefits be to you if you were able to reduce the chronic stress in your life?

What are the "costs" to you if you do not reduce chronic stress? (Examples: *more anxiety, weight gain, trouble sleeping*).

List 2-4 action steps that you will take to manage chronic stress in your life. (*Examples: seek assistance from a therapist, use a morning journal, start meditation practice*). **When you are ready, implement your Action Steps..**

Takeaways & Highlights

The path to thriving with a sugar-free lifestyle is about creating a balanced life based on three pillars of vibrant health: how we think, how we eat, and how we live.

How we live includes several components, including physical movement, restful sleep, and managing stress.

Physical Movement

Incorporating exercise into your daily routine provides a range of benefits, including clearing the blood of glucose, boosting insulin sensitivity, improving heart and cardiovascular health, and aiding your body in fat burning.

Exercise can be divided into several categories: Physical Activity, Aerobic Exercise, Recreational Activities, and Flexibility/Strength training.

Exercise Guidelines

- If you are under a doctor's care for any physical condition, clear any exercise program with your physician before starting.
- Start any new exercise routine slowly, with a gradual build up.
- Stop whenever you don't feel well
- Be consistent.
- Drink plenty of fluids.
- Make attentive foot care an integral part of your exercise program.

- Learn how your body responds to particular types of exercise by checking your blood glucose levels before, during, and after exercise.
- Know the symptoms of hypoglycemia.

Restful Sleep

Sleep deprivation raises levels of ghrelin, the hunger hormone, and decreases levels of leptin, the hormone that makes us feel full. To compensate for lower energy levels, people who sleep poorly may seek out high carbohydrate foods that actually drain our energy and cause roller-coaster blood sugar levels.

Tips for getting restful sleep

- Focus on controlling your blood sugar levels during the day and early evening.
- .Don't eat a heavy meal in the evening before bedtime.
- Moderate consumption of caffeine and alcohol.
- Limit the consumption of liquids 1-2 hours before going to bed.
- Set and maintain a consistent bedtime.
- Fall asleep in your bedroom, not on the sofa.
- Develop a bedtime ritual that includes relaxing activities.
- Create a peaceful, sleep-friendly environment.
- If you have concerns or adopting fundamental lifestyle changes doesn't improve your sleep, it's important to talk to your doctor. Your doctor can assess whether you have a more significant sleep issue, such as diabetic neuropathy, nighttime eating syndrome, or sleep apnea, and recommend further tests or treatment

Chronic Stress

How stress affects your body.

- A stressful event occurs (You step into the street, and a car turns the corner, almost hitting you).
- The body reacts to physical cues from the event (shallow breathing, heart racing, etc.)
- The hormones adrenalin and cortisol are released

- Cortisol quickly breaks down available sugars, fats and proteins in order to supply energy (providing the energy needed to get out of the street quickly to avoid being hit by the car).

Once the crisis is over, your body returns to its normal state.

When stress becomes chronic or unmanaged, the constant release of adrenaline and cortisol begins to have negative effects, including increased hunger, cravings, elevated blood sugar levels, and muscle tissue breakdown.

Tips for managing chronic stress in your daily life

Incorporate de-stressing activities daily.

- Practice deep breathing.
- Prioritize your health & take time for yourself.
- Exercise regularly.
- Write in a journal.
- Practice gratitude & enjoy life.
- Develop a support system.
- Eliminate added sugar and other trigger foods.

PHASE THREE:
Transform Your Mind to Stay Free from Sugar

- Find the Thoughts, Roadblocks, and Eating Patterns Getting in Your Way
- Reverse Sabotaging Thoughts, Habits, and Eating Patterns
- Eliminate Clutter in Your Space to Create an Environment that Supports Lasting Change
- Enjoy Life

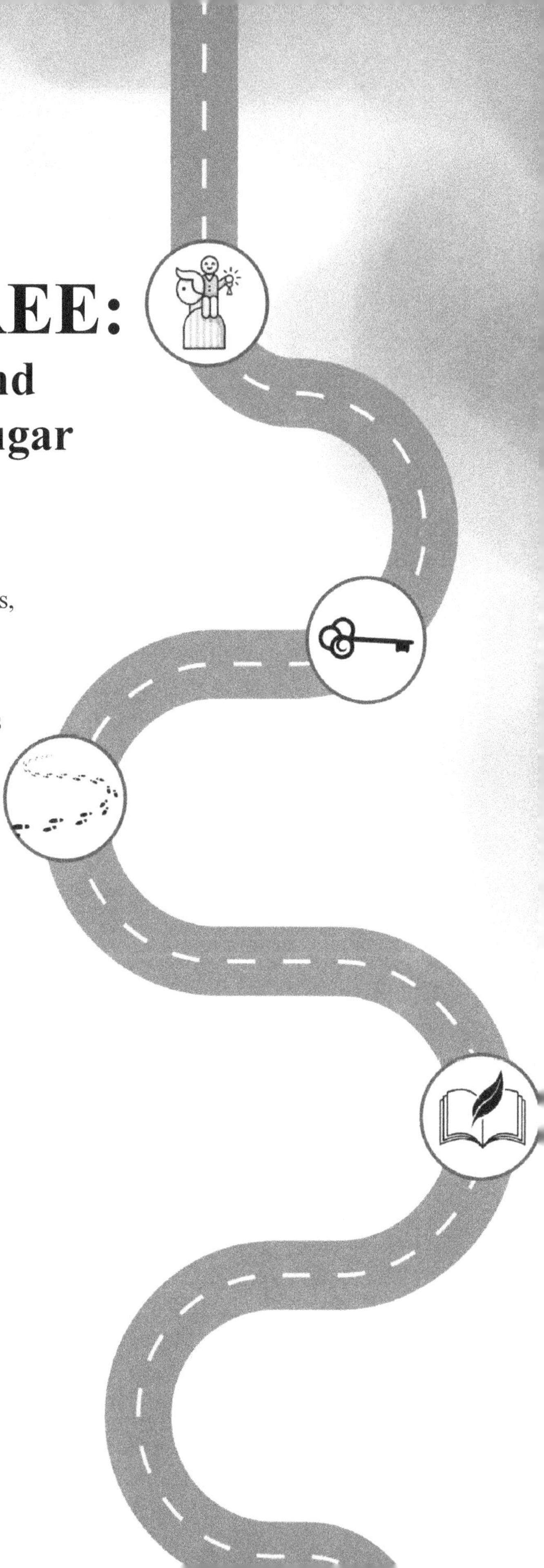

CHAPTER 15
Find the Thoughts, Roadblocks, and Eating Patterns Getting in Your Way

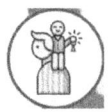

Coach on Your Shoulder

Phases 1 and 2 were focused on learning how to make lifestyle changes and the practical aspects of creating a sugar-free lifestyle. You have learned how to create a food plan and support it with exercise, restful sleep, and effective stress management.

For many, following a new food plan and eliminating sugar becomes a consistent way of life. Although it is not always easy, they find that their cravings have subsided, and with clear guidelines, they are able to stay on track for the long term. If this is you, the steps in Phase 3 will be the icing on the cake, with additional coaching and tips that will help you handle roadblocks when life gets in the way.

But for many, the path to living sugar-free is filled with challenges, and everyday eating is an overwhelming process. Do you struggle to quit sugar for the long term? If yes, one of the most important things you can do is gain clarity about the trigger foods that drive your continued desire for sweets and other foods that sabotage your efforts. The ultimate goal is to eliminate sugar and all trigger foods from your food consumption.

As you learned in Chapter 4 (Change Your Relationship to Sugar), the sensations and emotions that signal when you are full, hungry, or wanting to eat something like candy, ice cream, bread, or potato chips are the result of a complex combination of chemical reactions occurring in your body along with life circumstances and stimuli that drive your desire for sugar and other trigger foods.

There are many different types of stimuli that I refer to as trigger food motivators. It is only when you have clarity about why you reach for sugar and other trigger foods that you can change habits, thoughts, and behaviors to eliminate the trigger foods that take you off track. Phase 3 is designed to help you discover the stimuli/motivators underlying your cravings, as well as how to eliminate trigger foods by changing behaviors and daily habits.

This chapter will focus on identifying your trigger foods and the situations that motivate you to take that first bite, and you will use this information to change your habits in Chapter 16.

Key Concepts

Trigger Food Review

Many individuals initially do very well with their sugar-free lifestyle. Then, without warning, they find themselves consuming sugar, and they don't know why. The sense of being out of control makes them feel overwhelmed and sometimes hopeless.

If you have ever felt this way, the good news is that there is a straightforward solution for ending the struggle. First, you have to have clarity about which foods are your trigger foods, and then you need to identify and resolve the motivators that lead you to consume sugar or other trigger foods. The latter is achieved by having clarity about why specific motivators cause you to lose control and how you can establish new habits that help you make different choices.

As we learned in earlier chapters, trigger foods:

- Drive physical and/or emotional cravings for more of the same food, or
- Lead to cravings and binging on other foods.

Trigger foods act in our bodies in different ways, including:

- Causing fast/sharp spikes in both glucose and insulin, resulting in roller-coaster blood sugar levels, with peaks, crashes, and resulting cravings,
- Causing cravings due to an engineered combination of sugar, fat, salt, or other highly processed ingredients,
- Impacting hormones that regulate appetite (Insulin, Ghrelin, Leptin), leading to increased hunger, inability to stop eating, and
- Impacting Neurochemicals that direct our moods and survival functions (Serotonin, Dopamine, and Endorphins), causing imbalances that can lead to intense food cravings and increased desire for Trigger foods.

Whether a particular food triggers cravings and disordered eating depends on how the food affects your body, based on your unique biochemistry and other emotional factors and motivators. What is a trigger food for you might not be one for someone else. For example, many people can eat a cookie or two if it is made with non-grain-based flour and a natural sugar alternative. Not me! One cookie (of any kind) and I am, as they say, "off to the races". Cookies are a trigger food for me, primarily due to underlying emotional issues that I shared in my story, and I need to avoid them.

In Chapter 12, you listed your personal trigger foods as a first step towards eliminating them. In this chapter, you will gain clarity about the life situations and motivators that influence your food choices so that you can learn what you can do differently when confronting these motivators in the future.

If you still find yourself returning to sugar in any form, most likely, you have not yet fully addressed one or more of the stimuli/motivators described below that lead to consuming sugar and other trigger foods. It is almost impossible to eliminate trigger foods if you don't first identify why you reach for them.

Common Motivators for Consuming Trigger Foods

Various habits, situations, or emotions can be the initial stimuli leading to consuming a trigger food. Below is an overview of common motivators.

Busy Lifestyles and Need for Convenience:

Processed or convenience foods require less time and energy for food preparation. With our busy, sometimes overscheduled lives, seeking convenience foods to make food preparation easier is not unusual. The problem is that today, many convenience foods are what we call "ultra-processed" foods (UPFs) that contain added sugar (or other sugar sources) along with a combination of unhealthy fats, high levels of salt, and other food additives. When these elements are combined, they can cause blood sugar spikes and activate the brain's reward centers, releasing dopamine, a feel-good neurotransmitter that can lead to intense cravings for these foods.

Depending on your lifestyle, consuming convenience foods may be a necessary choice. It is not required to cut out all convenience or processed foods as long as they do not cause a sharp/fast rise in blood glucose levels and are not a trigger food for you. The key is to eliminate convenience foods that contain added sugar and other ingredients that cause cravings and lead to unwanted consumption of excess amounts of that particular food or other foods. Pre-cut and frozen vegetables, plain yogurt, bottled no-sugar salad dressings, canned beans, seasoning mixes, rotisserie chicken, low-carb wraps, and low-sodium prepared soups are just a few of the healthy convenience foods that can help make meal preparation faster and easier.

Sabotaging Learned Behaviors and Habits:

A habit is a routine behavior that is repeated regularly and generally occurs subconsciously. We all have habits that influence our food choices for meals and snacks. These habits often stem from our childhood or other family traditions, while some develop in adulthood as we navigate work and family life. Some habits lead you towards your health goals. Other habits are negative behaviors that sabotage efforts to live a sugar-free lifestyle. Break Free From the Sugar Blues aims to support you in forming positive habits that help you stay on track. Some common examples of habits that tend to sabotage efforts include:

- Eating a bagel or pastry every day for breakfast (at home or on the way to work)
- Ordering home fries and toast with eggs when eating breakfast at a restaurant
- Grabbing a quick sandwich with fries for lunch
- Skipping lunch and loading up on snacks in the late afternoon

- Drinking soda throughout the day at home or work
- Always including potatoes, rice, or pasta as a side dish with dinner
- Snacking on foods such as chips while watching TV

The good news is that once you are aware of habits that sabotage your sugar-free lifestyle, you can begin to put new habits in their place. In this chapter, you will focus on identifying the habits you want to change, and in Chapter 16, we will explore how to make positive lifestyle choices.

Life Situations

Controlling the food that comes into our home makes it more manageable to live a sugar-free lifestyle. A general rule for my home is "if you don't want to eat it, don't buy it or bring it home." If there are children or other adults who eat differently (including foods with added, natural or hidden sugars), it is more challenging, but still doable. For example, you can create separate locations where those foods are stored, and most importantly, develop a plan for yourself when others are eating foods you need to avoid.

But we can't always stay at home, and there are many situations where "life gets in the way," and we find ourselves face to face with sugar and trigger foods. Examples include family celebrations, birthday parties, eating at restaurants, funerals, office parties, outings with children or grandchildren, weddings, barbecues, and vacations.

When faced with these situations, it is not unusual to find ourselves going off track and indulging in foods we would not ordinarily consume. The most important thing you can do in these situations is to take care of yourself and your needs. You don't have to eat Aunt Mary's birthday cake to make her happy, you don't have to put your hamburger on a roll or eat potato salad at the family barbecue, and it is OK to ask your server to bring you oil and vinegar for your salad rather than the house dressing with sugar in it.

Becoming Too Hungry, Angry, Lonely, and/or Tired

HALT is an acronym for Hungry, Angry, Lonely, Tired. It's a tool used to remind people that these four common stressors can impair judgment and make it hard to stay away from sugar. Being hungry, angry, lonely, or tired does not mean you will always crave sugar. The problem comes when you become so intensely hungry, angry, lonely, or tired that you lose control of your ability to make conscious food choices, and you find yourself mindlessly or obsessively consuming sugar and other trigger foods.

If becoming too hungry, angry, lonely, or tired is an issue for you, it is crucial to recognize and alleviate the underlying situations that got you there so that you can address them proactively and avoid behaviors that could jeopardize your ability to stay on track. For example, when you have gone too long without eating and become too hungry, a subsequent drop in blood sugar can cause feelings of irritability that can be easily mistaken for a craving. In this instance, you can establish new habits to prevent going too long between meals. And if you do find yourself in a state of extreme hunger, rather than grab a candy bar, you can choose a healthy snack, such as a combination of protein and non-starchy carbohydrate, and see if it makes a difference. Your desire for sugar will likely wane once your body is nourished.

Emotional Eating:

Emotional eating, also known as stress eating, is the propensity to eat in response to positive and negative emotions. It involves using food to fill emotional needs, rather than eating to resolve hunger.

Indeed, most people occasionally want sugar-laden food as a pick-me-up, reward, or celebratory treat. For those who do not have an underlying issue with emotional eating, it is less challenging to avoid sugar in these situations or to stop eating sugar after a small indulgence. But when turning to sugar is your primary emotional coping mechanism, the daily act of eating can become a nightmare, leading to a cycle where the ability to avoid sugar often feels impossible, and after consuming even a small amount, you crave more and more.

An emotional connection to food is often the result of deep-seated issues that started in childhood or traumatic experiences that could have happened at any point in your life. Regardless of how it manifests, the first step is determining whether emotional or stress eating is driving your sugar cravings. Only then can you delve deeper into your particular issues so that you can begin to make conscious decisions about when, what, and how you eat, especially when emotional triggers come into play.

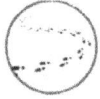

Action Steps

The questions and activities below are designed to help you identify the motivators that lead you to eat sugar and other trigger foods. If you need assistance, enlist a coach or friend to support you or participate in a peer support group. Sometimes it is helpful to use your daily journal to review the foods you eat and see if they are associated with any of the motivators listed.

In Chapter 16, we will discuss strategies for minimizing these motivators and implementing new behaviors to support you in eliminating trigger foods that sabotage your efforts.

Identify Motivators: Busy Lifestyles and Need for Convenience

	YES/NO
Do you regularly consume processed convenience foods that include added sugar or other trigger foods? (Do these convenience foods contain high amounts of natural sugar, hidden sugars such as grain-based flour, rice, potatoes, unhealthy fats, or large amounts of sodium?).	
Do you plan and shop regularly for convenience foods or are they a last-minute purchase?.	
Have you experienced times when a convenience or processed food led you to eat an excessive amount or binge on sugar or other foods?.	
Do any of the convenience/processed foods you consume cause fast/sharp rises in your blood sugar levels? (i.e. do you experience intense cravings or feel lethargic after eating or see the rise through blood testing or a CGM?)	

List the convenience/processed foods you consume that contain added sugar and/or are personal trigger foods in the space below. (If you started a list in Chapter 12, review it, and if you have updates, include them here.) In Chapter 16, we will explore meal planning techniques and shopping tips to help you eliminate convenience/processed trigger foods while taking into account your lifestyle and meal planning needs.

My list of convenience foods:

Identify Sabotaging Learned Behaviors and Habits

List the trigger foods you eat out of habit, and organize them according to the meals or snacks when you typically eat these foods. Include any specific activities that are habitual that are connected to eating trigger foods. Examples: Bagel or pastry for breakfast, snacks while watching TV, sandwich for lunch with chips, potatoes as a side dish with dinner, crackers or cookies before bed, specialty coffee drinks while out shopping, or soda at work.

(If you started a list in Chapter 12, review it. If you have updates, include them here.)

Breakfast:

Lunch:

Dinner:

Snacks:

Identify Motivators: Life Situations

When you find yourself in certain situations, such as holiday celebrations, barbecues, funeral gatherings, or birthday parties, are you more focused on the food than being present with the other attendees?

List the life situations that bring up habits, feelings, or emotions that lead you to eat trigger foods and the foods you commonly consume. (Examples: 1) Birthday Parties: Cake 2) Family Dinners (Mom's pasta dishes)

My List of Life Situations:

Identify Motivators: HALT

Are there times when you allow yourself to get too Hungry, Angry, Lonely, or Tired?

If you get into one of the HALT situations, does it lead you to eat sugar or foods you want to avoid?

If any of the HALT situations apply to you, provide a short description of what typically leads to this condition and a list of the trigger foods or foods with sugar you eat when you are too Hungry, Angry, Lonely, or Tired? (Example: Tired: I go to sleep too late at night, and the next day I find myself craving bread and other carbohydrates)

H (Hungry):

A (Angry):

L (Lonely):

T (Tired):

EMOTIONAL EATING

Do you reach for sugar (in any of its forms) in response to either negative or positive emotions, including stress eating?

List the emotions or stress conditions that lead you to sugar or other foods you want to avoid, and the trigger foods that you eat to manage emotions or stress. (Examples: 1) Worry: Cookies, Chocolate 2) Deadlines: Potato Chips, Soda, Chocolate

My List of Emotions, Stress Conditions, and Associated Trigger Foods:

Takeaways & Highlights

Trigger foods drive physical and/or emotional cravings for more of the same food or lead to cravings and binging on other foods.

Whether a particular food triggers cravings and disordered eating depends on how the food affects your body, based on your unique biochemistry and other emotional factors.

Trigger foods act in our bodies in different ways, including:

- causing fast/sharp spikes in both glucose and insulin, resulting in roller-coaster blood sugar levels, with peaks, crashes, and resulting cravings,
- causing cravings due to an engineered combination of sugar, fat, salt, or other highly processed ingredients,

- impacting hormones that regulate appetite (Insulin, Ghrelin, Leptin), leading to increased hunger, inability to stop eating, and
- impacting Neurochemicals that direct our moods and survival functions (Serotonin, Dopamine, and Endorphins), causing imbalances that can lead to intense food cravings & more desire for Trigger foods.

There is a difference between a trigger food and the motivation to take that first bite. Understanding this difference and developing habits to deal with your motivators puts you in the driver's seat and will help you eliminate trigger foods and stay on track.

Common motivators include:

- Busy Lifestyles and Need for Convenience
- Sabotaging Learned Behaviors and Habits
- Life Situations
- HALT (Hungry, Angry, Lonely, Tired)
- Emotional Eating

It is only when you have clarity about why you reach for sugar and other trigger foods that you can change habits, thoughts, and behaviors to eliminate the trigger foods that take you off track.

CHAPTER 16
Reverse Sabotaging Thoughts, Habits, and Eating Patterns

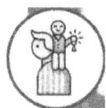

Coach on Your Shoulder

Congratulations! You have identified your trigger foods and the motivators that lead you to eat them. Now, you are ready to change sabotaging habits, behaviors, and pervasive thoughts so that you stop reaching for those foods and take charge of your sugar-free lifestyle.

Now is the time when the Four Elements of Change and Resilience discussed in Chapter 7 (Commitment, Connection, Consistency and Clarity) all come together to put you in the driver's seat for lasting change.

As you take action by establishing new habits, behaviors, and ways of thinking, remember that this is a process that requires patience and persistence. Knowing that making changes to eliminate trigger foods from your daily food plan takes time, don't be too hard on yourself. Life is always coming at you, and there will be times in the short term when you need to deal with situations where new habits may not yet be strong enough to make avoiding sugar and other trigger foods an automatic response. In the end of this chapter, in addition to taking steps for changing sabotaging habits, you will learn a STOP strategy for confronting sugar and moving on if you go off track.

We will also address emotional eating, so you can identify if it is an issue for you.

Key Concepts

Habits are the Fabric of Your Life

Once you have identified behaviors that are sabotaging your goals, the next step is putting new success habits in their place.

Success habits are repeated behaviors that eventually become automatic. Lasting change begins with daily behaviors that lead you toward your vision of health, and it is the little things you do every day that determine your success. The trick is to break down desirable behavior changes into manageable chunks, which I call success habits, that will ultimately become part of your daily routine.

It generally takes approximately 21 days to form a new habit and 90 days to turn that habit into a permanent lifestyle change. Initially, it is important to avoid drastic changes that lead to frustration. The key is to start implementing small new behaviors for a minimum of 21 days and to practice them for at least 90 days until they become a lasting, positive change.

How to Change a Habit

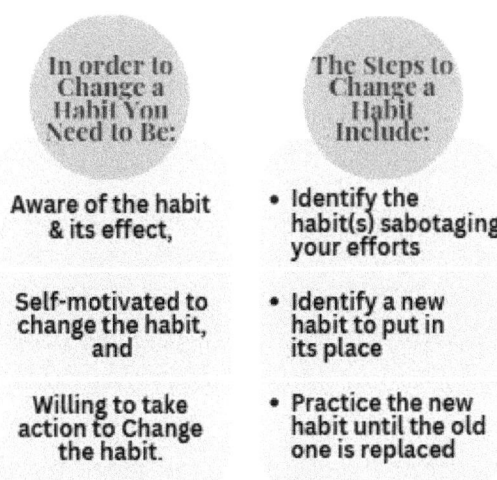

Your unique goals, biochemistry, and state of health will determine the changes you want to make, how many new habits you want to implement, how fast you want to go, and how long it will take for new habits to become lasting changes.

In the Taking Action portion of this chapter, you will begin to change or eliminate habits holding you back and establish new habits using the steps identified above.

Conquering Emotional Eating

As we discussed in earlier chapters, it is not unusual to seek out sugar or other comfort foods to cope or soothe difficult emotions. The problem arises when this coping mechanism becomes overused and a person consistently turns to trigger foods for comfort. In contrast to a person who is eating in response to a current, temporary stressor, emotional eaters are distinctly different. They eat to self-medicate and to numb unwanted feelings, usually those of anxiety, anger, fear or depression, and very often they are reacting to current situations through the lens of past, unresolved trauma.

Emotional eaters often seek out sugar-laden or salty, crispy foods such as cookies, cake, ice cream, specialty coffees or crunchy chips as their comfort food of choice. While the initial bite is pleasurable, the feeling of comfort is usually short-lived, especially hours later or the next day when guilt and self-loathing set in. The emotional eater is stuck in a vortex of painful eating that often starts with a need to self-medicate, then leads to eating trigger foods and the ultimate roller coaster ride of sugar highs followed by the inevitable lows, cravings, more food, and feelings of hopelessness.

My clients who deal with unmanaged emotional eating often ask me whether it ever gets better. My answer is absolutely yes, if you gain clarity about your trigger foods, identify your sabotaging habits and behaviors, and commit to consistently implementing new habits. Knowing your trigger foods and avoiding them will change your life. Will there be hard days? Also, absolutely, yes. That is life, but the truth is that you do not need to eat your way through it.

A starting point for managing emotional and stress eating is learning how to master control of your mind. You might be thinking OK, this is a little too 'woo-woo' for me. But stick with me.

Thoughts create our reality. Your emotional mind directly impacts your behavior, and every thought takes you towards or away from your vision of health. Numerous thought leaders have written about this subject, and it would be impossible to cover all of their theories in this book. The basic idea is that our thoughts determine our focus. And our thoughts also determine our emotions. Learn to control your thoughts, and you automatically control your focus and your feelings. The more aware you become, the more you can take responsibility for the thoughts and viewpoints you adopt and the choices you make. If emotional eating is driving a vicious cycle of eating sugar, it is possible for you to change your thoughts and begin to manifest change so that you can better manage emotional and stress eating.

The most common factors that impact stress and emotional eating are shown in the diagram below.

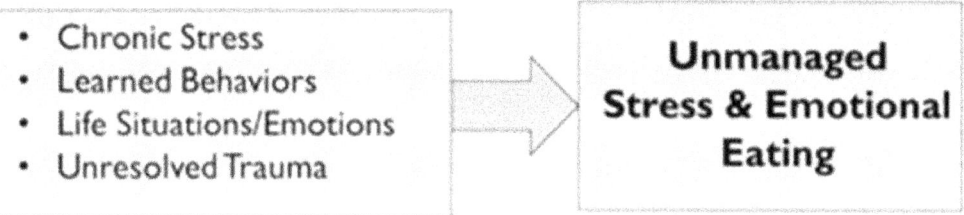

Two individuals whose theories are influential in popularizing theories about manifesting change through our thoughts are David Hawkins (the founder of the Map of Consciousness) and Esther and Jerry Hicks, who are most well known for their work in teaching and writing books about The Laws of Attraction.

David Hawkins is well known for developing a theory called The Map of Consciousness" that describes a range of emotions ranging from low to high frequencies (also referred to in his books as The Levels of Consciousness).

- The foundation of his teachings is that to experience positive change in your life and to experience vibrant health in all areas, you need to learn how to move from lower vibration emotions (Examples: shame, guilt, grief, fear, worry,

anxiety and anger) to higher vibration emotions such as courage, acceptance, willingness, love, joy, peace, gratitude, and generosity.
- He has many quotes attributed to him on this subject. One that sums up his philosophy is that "you get to choose what you focus upon, and you get to choose what manifests, and you get to choose how you feel about it when it does."

The ideas of Hawkins went mainstream through the teachings of Esther and Jerry Hicks, who are most well known for their work about "The Laws of Attraction." Like Hawkins, the Hicks teach that our thoughts manifest our reality, and the emotional energy that you put out into the world will be mirrored back to you in the form of external circumstances in your life.

It is not necessary to embrace the Laws of Attraction to conquer emotional eating. However, I invite you to take this opportunity to become more aware of the emotional energy you put into the world and to consider that it will be mirrored back to you in the form of external circumstances in your life. Put another way, you are the creator of your own experience. Your life experience is unfolding in response to what you think and how you view and respond to your reality.

In the Action Steps, you will explore a series of suggestions for connecting the dots between thoughts and emotions that lead to emotional eating. It is possible to incorporate habits that minimize the thoughts that lead to emotional eating and maximize daily thinking that helps you to make better food choices. However, the suggestions in this chapter do not replace seeking needed professional attention or identifying the underlying causes of emotional eating.

If you are experiencing anxiety, depression, or an eating disorder that requires professional care, seek assistance from a mental health care provider. If you are experiencing extreme depression or having suicidal thoughts, seek help from a professional ASAP.

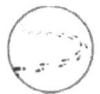

Action Steps

Begin The Process Of Choosing New Habits You Would Like to Implement By Reviewing Options and Identifying Those That Resonate With You.

To this point, you have identified your trigger foods (including added sugar) and considered what motivates you to eat them. Based on your answers to questions in Chapter 15 it is time to select a few initial behaviors and habits you would like to change and develop a game plan for replacing them with new habits and behaviors.

You will begin by becoming familiar with various habits you may want to implement. Don't worry if none resonate with you or if you choose one from each category or all of the options. For now, all you need to do is go through the lists in each of the five categories and identify success habits that appeal to you based on your needs and priorities.

The purpose of your habit checklist is to provide you with a roadmap of habits that will lead to lasting change. However, you don't want to set yourself up for failure by trying to do too many things at once. At the end of this section, there is an exercise where you will select a few new habits to start with that are a high priority or that you feel most confident about implementing.

You can continue implementing new success habits as you become more comfortable with your initial changes. After a few months, you will be surprised at how far you have come by being consistent with small daily action steps.

Success Habits for Managing Busy Lifestyles and Need for Convenience

Place a checkmark in the column next to the suggestions that resonate with you.

If you have children or other family members who eat foods that are triggers for you, find a separate location for these foods that you can avoid or work with them to try substitutes that work for everyone.
Plan 3-5 meals and create a shopping list to create those meals along with snacks and other basics needed for the week
Keep a well-stocked refrigerator, freezer, and pantry so you can create an easy meal or snack at any time. (This does not mean overbuy, but have the basics on hand to avoid constantly ordering out or eating highly processed junk food)
Use sugar-free and low-processed convenience foods such as frozen vegetables, meats, and packaged meals wisely when it makes sense to make your life easier.
If you only need a few items, write them down and stick to the list. Do not impulse shop.
Pick a day to make a portion of your meals ahead of time, such as preparing a casserole, chili, or hearty soup.
Do not shop when you are hungry. Eat something before going to the store or bring a bottle of water to sip while shopping.
Use containers to store cut-up vegetables, mini-snack trays, or portioned side dishes.
Use recipes as inspiration. Become comfortable with substituting ingredients or making a portion of the recipe with a convenience food rather than starting everything from scratch. (exception: baked goods)
Prepare foods that can be frozen and eaten throughout the week.
Invest in cooking tools designed to make it easier to prepare food quickly and deliciously. (examples: high speed blender, mini-mandolin, toaster/air fryer combo, table-top indoor grill)
Do not bring foods with added sugar or other trigger foods into the house. (See the suggestion below if you have children or other family members who eat foods that trigger you.)

More Ideas for Changing Convenience Food Habits

Preparing food at home does not have to be time-consuming or complicated. Here are some tips for fitting food preparation into your schedule.

Keep it Simple: It is fun to find interesting recipes and create a gourmet meal. But, if you want to eat at home more often, consider designating one night to try new things or make a more complex meal, and keep the menus for the rest of the week simple. When eating simply, try to make your meal visually pleasing by using pretty plates or serving bowls and be aware of not just how your food tastes but how it looks. A beautiful plate or bowl of simple foods appeals to all of your senses and is highly satisfying when eaten slowly and mindfully.

Use the "almost from scratch method" to prepare meals and snacks: For example, if a recipe calls for shredded chicken, start with a pre-cooked rotisserie chicken rather than cooking chicken breasts from scratch. A rotisserie chicken is a great starting point for soups, stews, stir-fry dishes, salads, chicken salad, or to make low-carb roll-ups or tacos. You can purchase a whole pre-cooked chicken from most stores, but if you're concerned about the ingredients, you can also pick a day to roast your own and have it available for dishes throughout the week.

Some other ideas include using bottled marinades, starting with canned seasoned beans for chili, using prepared bone broth and pre-cut or frozen vegetables for soups or side dishes, and combining prepared salad mixes with fresh vegetables to add variety and cut down on cutting time.

Food items that I always keep on hand to make quick meals and snacks include sugar free sauces and marinades, low carb wraps, canned artichoke hearts, canned beans, frozen vegetables and berries, good quality cheese, cooked quinoa in pouches, baked tofu, chicken broth, olives, hummus, pre-made dips, and pre-cut vegetables.

Plan and Prep Ahead: Prepping food one day a week is another way to make weekly mealtimes easier and avoid reliance on convenient trigger foods. Start by picking a day that works into your schedule to try some of the ideas below.

- Cut vegetables like broccoli, cauliflower, carrots or zucchini and put them into containers to save time prep time later in the week.
- Prepare a jar of picked red onions for salads or a batch of caramelized onions for stir-fries, omelets, or quinoa dishes.
- Press cabbage for snacks, salads, stir-fries, and other dishes.
- Cook a pot of quinoa that can serve as a base for a vegetable/protein bowl or side dish.
- Use a Dutch Oven or crockpot to cook soup, stews, chili, or meatballs that can be used throughout the week. I often prepare a big batch of meatballs in my crockpot that can be eaten with spaghetti squash, topped with ricotta and melted

cheese in a meatball parmesan bowl, or mashed and eaten as sloppy joes over savory chaffles.

- Prepare a meatloaf or tofu loaf that can be eaten with sides or sliced up for sandwiches later in the week.
- Roast a pan of vegetables that can be added to stir-fries and soups or eaten as a side dish. The vegetables that I typically roast in the fall and winter include butternut and acorn squash, brussels sprouts, cauliflower, broccoli, onions, and carrots. In the spring and summer, I like to add asparagus, peppers, and zucchini to my roasting trays.
- Cook full meals ahead of time, like food service delivery companies, and freeze them to use as needed.

Keep foods on hand to prepare mini cheese, charcuterie, or mezze plates: There are many nights when I'm running late or don't feel like cooking. Putting together a beautiful plate that combines items from my fridge and pantry solves the problem and provides a satisfying meal. I often create plates with themes such as:

- Italian with meats, cheeses, olives, peppers, and dips.
- Greek with hummus, tabbouleh, olives, feta and Greek salad.
- Japanese with deconstructed sushi on a plate.
- Mexican with bean salad, guacamole, lettuce, and grain-free low-carb nachos.

Stock your pantry with basics: A well-stocked pantry can reduce stress by ensuring that you have essential ingredients available for quick meal planning, improvising with recipes, and avoiding last-minute grocery trips. You will find ideas in the next Chapter that includes how to create your own Kitchen Pantry Makeover.

Have the tools you need to make cooking easier: Certain kitchen tools can make a big difference. The equipment and tools that I rely on include:

- Crock Pot and Dutch Oven. Nothing makes it easier to put a delicious meal on the table than concocting stews, soups, chili, and all sorts of protein dishes ahead of time in a crockpot or Dutch Oven.
- Handheld Mandolin. Want to make a cucumber salad or slice other vegetables in 5 minutes? A small handheld mandolin is the answer. Mandolin blades are

very sharp, so you have to be careful when you get down to the end of the vegetable you are slicing (I wear a protective glove specially made to protect fingers when cutting & slicing)

- High-Speed Blender. I use mine every day for smoothies, but my blender gets a workout for more than that. Have leftover roasted vegetables? Throw them in a high-speed blender with some chicken broth and seasonings (cream is optional) and enjoy a fabulous soup. A Vitamix blender has the extra benefit of having a very high speed that warms the soup, so no cooking is necessary.
- Air Fryer. I purchased a brand that also takes the place of your toaster and has a built-in convection oven and dehydrator. You can "air fry" vegetables instead of roasting them, prepare succulent chicken and fish, and cook a whole host of foods in just minutes, without a lot of oil or butter.
- Indoor Grill. I love my small indoor electric grill. Marinating fish and throwing it on the grill could not be easier, and it always comes out great. Ditto for grilled chicken. I slice chicken breasts into strips, marinate them, cook them on the grill, and I have chicken for the week to eat in salads, stir fries or on their own for a quick lunch. It is easy, fast, and updated copper lined grills make clean up a breeze.

Think Outside the Box: In the past, meals had specific routines associated with them. Breakfast was eggs, oatmeal or cereal. Lunch was usually a sandwich or salad. Dinner typically was a protein (consisting of chicken, meat or fish) with a side of carbohydrates (usually some potatoes or rice or pasta combined with a small serving of vegetables. Sometimes, the meal started with a soup or salad.

Today, I don't have any specific rules for meals, except to try to base them on non-starchy vegetables, healthy proteins, and healthy fats. Other than that, I sometimes have a bowl of bone broth with vegetables, leftover salmon, or a salad for breakfast. Lunch is often a smoothie with lots of protein, and to keep things simple, I end the day with a stir fry or mezze platter for dinner. Some nights I also like to have "breakfast for dinner," and I might prepare a frittata or vegetable/cheese omelet paired with my favorite chaffle.

Whether you are cooking just for yourself or for children or other family members who may have different likes and needs, keeping it simple, and having the tools you need will make mealtime more manageable and help you to lessen your reliance on highly processed, triggering, convenience foods.

Success Habits for Changing Sabotaging Learned Behaviors

In the tables below, place a checkmark in the column next to the suggestions that resonate with you.

<u>New Breakfast Habits</u>

Combine protein with carbohydrates (including vegetables, if possible) that minimize fast/sharp spikes in blood sugar levels	
Avoid high glycemic fruit (small amounts of berries are OK)	
If you like to stop at a coffee shop, such as Starbucks, choose a breakfast option with protein, such as egg bites, to have with your coffee.	
Make a batch of chaffles to have during the week or make your own egg bites	

<u>New Lunch Habits:</u>

If you like having a sandwich or burger, substitute a low-carb wrap or lettuce wrap for the bread.	
Replace fries or chips with pickles, coleslaw, vegetables (raw or cooked), soup, or salad. Or substitute sweet potato fries for traditional fries	
Make a batch of chaffles to have during the week or make your own egg bites	
Have a bowl of soup or chili instead of a sandwich (add in a salad or a side of protein or vegetables if you want a heartier meal)	
Drink water or iced tea instead of soda.	

<u>New Dinner Habits:</u>

Avoid rice, potatoes, and pasta. Plan dinner meals around protein, non-starchy vegetables, and healthy fats (minimize consumption of starchy vegetables or foods with "hidden" sugar and high glycemic fruit)	
Use sugar-free and low-processed convenience foods such as frozen vegetables, meats, and packaged meals wisely when you need to make your life easier.	
Enjoy a cheese platter with a small amount of low-glycemic fruit or a cup of tea or coffee after a meal instead of a sweet dessert.	

New Snack Habits:

Remove trigger foods that you consume as snacks from your home (and/or workplace)
Keep a separate snack food location for children or others that you live with (for snack foods containing sugar or your trigger foods)
Be prepared at home and at work with no-sugar snack foods that do not create fast/sharp rise in your blood sugar levels.
Stop eating after 8 PM (a late night meal on occasion is OK, but it should not be the norm)

New Habits for All Meals and Snacks

Slow down, eat mindfully, and savor your food.
Eat sitting down in an environment that helps you to eat more mindfully.
Do not overfill your plate, and watch portion sizes.
Learn to recognize when you feel full and do not eat past this point.

Success Habits For Avoiding Trigger Foods in Life Situations

Humans are inherently social beings, and food often plays a central role in our social lives, from celebrations and holidays to family gatherings and social events. When you are trying to avoid sugar and other trigger foods, many life situations can be stressful. My clients want to know, "How can I stay healthy during special occasions when faced with food and the underlying stress of trying to avoid sugar and other trigger foods?" Here are some suggestions and guidelines for getting through life situations with your sugar-free lifestyle intact. Overall, the best advice I can give is to be gentle with yourself. Reach out for support when you need it, and enjoy everything your special events have to offer.

Place a checkmark in the column next to the suggestions that resonate with you.

Be prepared and eat something before your event.   Before going to a restaurant, party, or any special occasion, eat something ahead of time so that you don't arrive starving and dive right into bread, chips, or other

triggering foods. Try pairing hummus or bean dip with raw vegetables. A bowl of soup is another healthful option

Bring a dish that you can share to avoid consuming trigger foods.
If you are invited to someone's home for a meal or celebration, everyone will appreciate a tasty addition to their party table. I always bring one thing that I know I will be able to eat and that everyone else will enjoy. It depends on the event. For dinners, I usually bring a vegetable dish like delicious Brussels sprouts with caramelized onions -- or for a buffet, I love to bring a beautiful array of grilled or roasted vegetables.

Ask for what you need.
If your special occasion is at a restaurant, it takes resolve to avoid a bread basket. If you are feeling tempted, when the waiter is taking drink orders, ask to have a salad or soup brought out right away so that you have something to eat while others are eating bread. Also, when you order your meal, even if it comes with a starch that you don't want, you can ask to have extra vegetables in its place. Don't feel embarrassed about asking questions or making Evaluate a buffet table before digging in: Buffets are the ultimate minefield for anyone trying to avoid sugar and tempting trigger foods. A good strategy is to observe the entire buffet before putting anything on your plate. Find the items that fit into your food plan and fill your plate with those first. Enjoy your selections, and if you find yourself obsessing over a trigger food on the buffet table, order a cup of coffee or tea rather than returning to the buffet to select a trigger food. If a buffet of desserts is offered, proceed to the next suggestion.

Take care of your sweet tooth.
When sweets are part of a celebration or offered on a lavish buffet table, with some strategies in place, you can get through it without feeling deprived. First and foremost, return to tip #1, and eat something before the event. That way, your blood sugars won't be all over the place, and you will be less likely to crave sweets. Another way to avoid eating desserts loaded with sugar is to bring along a sweet indulgence to enjoy. I always carry a few pieces of stevia or monk fruit sweetened dark chocolate in my purse. When faced with a dessert buffet, cookies at the office, or party desserts, I bring out my chocolate, have some tea or coffee, and I am good to go. Maybe I will have a bite or two of whatever else is being offered, but with my treat in hand, I don't feel deprived, and I am much less likely to eat an amount that will wreak havoc on my blood sugars.

Get enough rest and keep up your exercise.
When you are tired, you begin to crave more carbohydrates, especially bread, cookies and sweets to keep your energy up. So make sure that you are giving your body the rest it needs. If possible, try to keep up with your exercise routine. You will have more energy and avoid holiday/party remorse by staying on track.

Success Habits to Avoid Being Too Hungry, Angry, Lonely or Tired

Each of the HALT states can negatively affect mood, behavior, and decision-making capabilities, potentially leading to relapse or unhelpful coping mechanisms. Regularly checking in with yourself by asking, "Am I becoming too hungry, angry, lonely, or tired?" can significantly enhance self-awareness. Recognizing these states early allows you to address your needs proactively, preventing emotional spirals and promoting physical and emotional wellness.

Becoming too hungry or too tired is typically related to the physical state of your body, while the states of anger and loneliness are more closely tied to underlying emotions that can lead to emotional eating. Anger is a strong emotion that many of us have experienced in situations where we hesitate to confront others or avoid sticking up for ourselves. We fear conflict or worry about hurting relationships, so instead, we internalize our feelings, harboring hurt and resentment. These feelings often manifest in frustration, anger, and eventually, self-sabotaging emotional eating of sugar and other comfort foods.

Below are four coaching tips to help you gain clarity around the four HALT motivators and start implementing new habits.

- **Acknowledge and learn to recognize your feelings**. When you feel hungry, angry, lonely, or tired, recognizing your physical or emotional state is the first step toward effectively managing both your emotions and actions. Are you currently aware when you are feeling any of these states? If yes, that is a significant first step. If no, take time to become more in tune with your physical and emotional state, such as practicing the STOP exercise when you find yourself craving sugar or other trigger foods.
- **Write in a journal**. Expressing your feelings in writing can be a therapeutic outlet for exploring and connecting with your emotions without fear of judgment or confrontation.
- **Develop a plan for each of the four states of HALT**. Use the new habit suggestions below to take action and avoid sugar and other trigger foods.

- **Seek Support.** If you feel stuck or the situation(s) you face are too much to handle alone, talk to a trusted friend or therapist who can offer perspective, validation, and guidance.

In the tables below relating to HALT, place a checkmark in the column next to the suggestions that resonate with you.

Habits to Avoid Being Too Hungry

Maintain a regular eating schedule	
Be prepared and keep sugar-free snacks that are not personal trigger foods easily accessible.	
Stay hydrated, as thirst can sometimes mimic hunger	
Eat enough at meals to satisfy your hunger (for example, don't choose to eat a small lettuce salad to avoid calories only to find yourself ravenous an hour later)	
To sustain energy and avoid roller-coaster blood sugar levels, include foods rich in protein, fiber, and healthy fats.	
Use the STOP method if you find yourself hungry and reaching for sugar or trigger foods	

Habits to Proactively Manage Anger

Use deep breathing techniques when feeling overwhelmed.	
Seek professional counseling or anger management workshops if anger frequently feels unmanageable. Seek help identifying the source of your anger and techniques to manage your emotions.	
Engage in regular physical activity to reduce stress and release pent-up tension.	
Practice mindfulness and meditation.	
Acknowledge your feelings and write in your journal.	
When possible, speak up respectfully to address a tense situation.	
Use the STOP method if you find yourself angry and reaching for sugar or trigger foods.	

Habits to Avoid Becoming Too Lonely

It is possible to feel alone even in a room full of people or when you are physically by yourself. The suggestions below are designed to help you feel more connected, reduce your sense of isolation, and find ways to become more involved with others through social interaction.

Make a plan to include a daily activity that gets you out of the house and around other people, such as taking a walk in a public park, exploring a museum, visiting a library, or browsing through books at your local bookstore. Getting out and around others can lift your spirits even if you are not technically engaging in social interactions.
Find and attend a class that interests you in a local adult night school or other community center.
Join a group that has participants with similar interests or that are working on issues that you can relate to. This could include support groups or group therapy sessions.
When you feel lonely at home, fill your space with music to lift your spirits. If the mood strikes, dance along to engage your body and mind.
Find solo hobbies and activities that you enjoy doing on your own, such as reading, painting, yoga, or a new activity that you have been wanting to try.
Reach out and connect with friends and family members. If they are open to it, make a date to get together for an activity such as a meal, movie, or cup of coffee/tea. Try to schedule a meeting time. Open-ended plans to catch up sometime in the future often never materialize.
Volunteer and participate with others in an organization where you can meet and interact with people with a mutual passion for helping others
Consider getting a pet, fostering a dog or cat, or if that's not feasible, volunteering at an animal shelter.
Use the STOP method if you find yourself very lonely and reaching for sugar or trigger foods to ease how you are feeling.

Habits to Get Enough Sleep and Avoid Being Too Tired

Don't eat a heavy meal in the evening before bedtime.
Moderate consumption of caffeine and alcohol.
Limit the consumption of liquids 1-2 hours before going to bed.
Set and maintain a consistent bedtime

Fall asleep in your bedroom, not on the sofa	
Develop a bedtime ritual that includes relaxing activities.	
Create a peaceful, sleep-friendly environment	

Success Habits to Conquer Emotional Eating

In the tables below relating to conquering emotional eating, place a checkmark in the column next to the suggestions that resonate with you.

Habits To Manage Daily Thoughts that Impact Emotional Eating

Get support from a coach, therapist, group, or individuals, such as family or friends, if you still find yourself overwhelmed with feelings leading to emotional eating.	
Use a daily journal to document your feelings, stay on track, and take action.	
Clean and organize your environment.	
Exercise and spend time in nature.	
Celebrate your accomplishments.	
Focus on progress and growth.	
Acknowledge your feelings.	
Use a worry jar to release worries.	
Forgive yourself and others.	
Meditate.	
Learn to Silence Your Inner Critic.	
Surround Yourself with Positive People.	

Habits To Experience More Peace, Love, and Joy

Practice gratitude.	
Visualize your dreams.	
Give and receive love.	
Enjoy your journey.	

Spend time with people who you love.
Listen to your favorite music.

Habits For More Acceptance, Willingness and Courage:

Create your vision
Develop goals and an action plan.
Gain clarity about your vision and purpose.
Volunteer.
Perform random acts of kindness.
Compliment others.
Give someone a hug.

How to Use a Worry Jar to Manage Fear, Worry, and Anxiety

A few years ago, I was shopping for a birthday card for my granddaughter when I came across a little box with a quote that spoke about not stressing over things we cannot control. It reminded me of a technique that has been extremely helpful to me and my clients for putting worries aside, and in turn, calming reactive eating that can occur when worry gets the best of us.

Worry is a common denominator among most stress eaters. Many of us tend to worry about things that may never happen, and if they do, we are very often able to handle them. If you are grappling with worry and resulting stress eating, just for today, start by committing to not worrying about things you can't control.

NEXT, hand your "worries" over to the universe. Write each thing you are worried about on a separate small piece of paper. Fold your worry entries, place them in a jar or box, and mentally release them. (I have several pretty jars and containers that I use for this purpose)

At the end of the week, take out the notes and review them to see 1) if they have resolved themselves or if they are still a "worry," and 2) if there is concrete action that you could be taking to address the situation. If the worry has been resolved throw it away. If it is not yet handled, take any useful positive actions and put the worry back in the box, letting go of what you cannot control.

And while you are letting go of your worries, make a list of 10 things you would rather do than eat when worry strikes, and put it on your fridge, your nightstand, or somewhere else where you can refer to it. (My list includes take a hot shower, play with my cat, sip tea, read my favorite magazines, ZOOM with my grandchildren, watch a favorite movie....you get the idea)

This process of letting go of what you can't control and taking action on the things, you can, eases both the worry and the intense reaction to soothe our nerves with food. I love the quote about worry below by Edith Armstrong, and putting my worries into a worry box is my version of keeping my mind open to positive thoughts and outcomes. (When the worries are in my box, they can't reach my number.)

I keep the telephone on my mind open to peace, harmony, health, love and abundance. Then, whenever doubt, anxiety, or fear try to call me, they keep getting a busy signal, and soon they forget my number. Edith Armstrong

On the flip side of keeping a "worry jar" it is also uplifting to keep a gratitude jar or journal. Practicing gratitude means taking the time to appreciate and be thankful for the good things in your life. This can increase your happiness and well-being, improving your relationships, and helping you to cope with stress and difficult situations.

You can incorporate gratitude into your daily routine by taking a moment to reflect on the things you are grateful for before bed or first thing in the morning. Practicing gratitude is a habit that takes time and effort, but it can have a powerful impact on your life.

Select a Few Habits to Incorporate Into Your Daily Routine

Pick a few habits to work on that have the highest priority, and then you can add more as you feel more comfortable with your new routines. Some habits will be performed weekly or intermittently throughout the week or month, such as picking a day to prep foods for use during the week. Others will be daily habits, such as not eating after 8 pm.

How to Use a Habit Tracker

One helpful method to provide motivation and visual feedback is to use a habit tracker in conjunction with the journaling techniques you learned in Chapter 13 (Validate, Monitor, and Adjust Your Plan). A habit tracker is a visual tool that helps you track your progress and stay motivated while you wait for the long-term rewards of your efforts to accumulate. You can use a habit tracker for daily, weekly or monthly routines.

The benefits of using a habit tracker in addition to a daily journal include:

- Creating a daily visual set of cues that remind you to act.
- Providing immediate feedback that shows you are on the right path.
- Encouraging you to stick with the habit and achieve consistency.
- Helping to improve clarity and insight into your patterns and behavior.
- Providing both motivation and accountability to stay on track.

There are many different tools and formats for tracking progress using a Habit Tracker. The easiest is to get a calendar or use a Habit Tracker Journal designed explicitly for developing new habits. There are also habit-tracking applications for those who prefer an automated approach.

To use the written Habit Tracker provided below, place a check in the circle for each day that you successfully implement your new habit. Start with the first circle and move through the circles for 21 days. If you missed a day, leave a blank circle and place a check the next time you complete performing the habit.

For example, if you practice deep breathing on Monday, Wednesday, and Friday, each of those dates gets an X. As time rolls by, the calendar or Habit Tracker template becomes a record of your habit streak. Placing an X or a Check Mark on each day is the classic look. If you want to adopt a more visual approach, you can shade in the cells in your habit tracker.

If possible, record each measurement immediately after the habit occurs. The completion of the habit is the cue to write it down.

If you miss one daily habit, try to get back into your routine as quickly as possible. The first time you miss a new habit does not need to send you into a downward spiral. Avoid negative self-talk that says your have failed, and instead pat yourself on the back for taking control of your actions and get back on your sugar-free path.

If you have identified a habit that you are finding particularly hard to change, use the STOP method to overcome the issues holding you back.

21 DAY HABIT TRACKER

Write the new habit you have committed to in the box below, along with any notes or activities you have identified to help you perform this habit.

Place an X in the circles below on each day that you put your new habit into place. If you miss a day, leave a blank circle and place a check the next time you perform the habit
START DATE:

Sunday	Monday	Tuesday	Wednesday	Thursday	Friday	Saturday
○	○	○	○	○	○	○
○	○	○	○	○	○	○
○	○	○	○	○	○	○
○	○	○	○	○	○	○

Use the STOP Technique When Life Gets in the Way

Changing habits and sabotaging behaviors is a process. In the beginning, it is not unusual to have a strong desire to change a behavior, yet still find yourself repeating old patterns. That is why it is critical to have a strategy you can use immediately while you are working on building new habits for your future.

Below is a method often referred to as "STOP" that slows down the action when you are eating or about to eat sugar or another trigger food so that you can step back and gain more clarity about the link between your thoughts, feelings, and the behavior you are facing right in the moment.

This allows you to connect with the inner voice that can guide you toward making better choices. The next time you find yourself reaching for a cookie, about to open a bag of potato chips, or standing in front of a buffet table ready to dive into the potato salad or desserts, try using the steps below to stop the action and give yourself a change to make the best decision in the moment.

- Step Outside of Yourself
- Trace Your Current Action Back to the Motivator
- Observe Your Thoughts and Clarify Your Actions
- Put a New Behavior in Place of the Old Behavior

Step Outside of Yourself. When you are faced with a situation that brings out thoughts and behaviors that you know are sabotaging your health, literally take a break in the "action" and take a look at what you are doing as if you are an impartial observer. This does two things. First, it changes the event from an unconscious behavior that is seemingly beyond your control to one that can be changed. Second, at a practical level, it slows you down so that you can choose some options.

For example, let's imagine that at the end of a long work day, you come through your front door and find yourself standing in front of an open cabinet, with a box of crackers in your hands, ready to binge on the entire box. On auto-pilot, you eat the first cracker as if in a trance.

Using the **STOP** method, the goal in this situation would be to consciously stop what you are doing for a moment so that you can set the stage for taking another course of action. Observe yourself right then as if you are a stranger watching a scene from a movie.

- What is your physical state? (how is your breathing, heartbeat, other physical sensations) Are you standing or sitting? Have you taken your coat off?
- Look at the crackers. What kind are they? How do they taste? Did you get a plate or are you just eating them quickly out of the box?

Now that you have slowed down the action, you are ready to take the next step.

Trace Your Current Action Back to the Motivator (that led you to your trigger food). Think back about what occurred that got you to this point. In other words, trace your current action back to the motivator that led you to open the cabinet and reach for the box of crackers.

Was it any of the motivators that we discussed so far? Convenience, Habit, HALT, Life Situation, or Emotional/Stress eating. Maybe it was a combination of one or more of these motivators.

In this situation, let's imagine that you ate a healthy breakfast and lunch, and you had a small snack of nuts and low-fat cheese around 3:00. So, as you reflect upon the situation, physically, there is no reason for you to be ravenous.

Thinking back, you remember that your boss took credit for some work that you did, and this is something that happens on a pretty regular basis. (not just to you but to everyone in the department) But, you didn't say anything about it. Instead, you "stewed" about it all afternoon, and by the time you got home you were angry and your emotions were "eating away at you."

Tracing your current action back to events that stimulated your current action is crucial because it enables you to uncover what is motivating your behavior and to clarify your thinking. It is a powerful technique that creates the opportunity to ask yourself questions that will reveal whether eating to calm yourself down is in your best interest and to brainstorm about new behaviors that can be put its place.

Observe Your Thoughts and Clarify Your Actions. Bringing conscious awareness to your choices opens the door to an honest self-assessment where you can ask yourself questions that will clarify the consequences of your actions.

Through this process, you gain clarity your choices and whether your actions support or sabotage your vision of health and well-being.

In this case if you are able to see that you were angry and were attempting to push your feelings down with food, you are in a better position to make a change in your behavior so that you can learn to address anger in a way that does not involve compulsive eating of sugar and other foods that sabotage your sugar-free lifestyle.

Mindless eating at the end of a long work day is actually quite common, although the motivation varies based on individual circumstances. For some of my clients, reaching for comfort foods at the end of their workday is the result of not eating enough during the day and letting themselves get too hungry. For others, it is a longstanding unconscious reaction to feelings such as exhaustion or anxiety. Regardless of the circumstances, once you can step back and identify the root causes and the choices you made in response to the circumstance, you are ready to take action steps to make a change.

Put a New Behavior in Place of the Old Behavior. The ultimate goal is to get yourself off autopilot and to gain clarity about the choices you make on a daily basis so that you can replace sabotaging habits with new behaviors.

Often, by the time you reach this step, you are able to put the box of crackers away and move on to taking a different approach, such as taking a walk, drinking a cup of tea, or making dinner.

If you find that you still ate a bunch of crackers, don't beat yourself up. Now that you have more clarity, you can brainstorm to identify alternative behaviors that provide options for responding to situations in a way that supports your well-being.

When you are eating as a response to feeling angry, some empowering questions might include:

- What can I do to deal with my anger in a way that does not harm me? (Get up from my desk and take a walk, find a quiet spot to do some deep breathing, share my feelings with a trusted person, or write in a journal.)
- What can I do to make sure that I have something healthy and ready to eat if I am not feeling 100 percent when I get home from work? (Shop on Sundays and

keep healthy food choices easily accessible. - Examples: cut up vegetables and hummus, salad with condiments, roasted sliced chicken breast, low fat cheese, or vegetable soup.)
- What can I do to resolve my issues around anger and emotional eating? (Seek assistance from a therapist or life coach, write in my journal, or explore beliefs that may be at the core using food to cope with anger)

NOW, close your eyes and visualize yourself engaging in the new behavior. How does it feel?

Finally, select some of the new behavior alternatives and practice putting them into action.

You may not be able to control the behaviors of others, but you can control your reactions and the choices you make that will ultimately either sabotage your efforts or lead you toward better health. With repetition, you will internalize new behaviors, and with practice, they will become automatic over time.

Takeaways & Highlights

Success habits are repeated behaviors that eventually become automatic. The trick is to break down desirable behavior changes into manageable chunks, which I call success habits, that will ultimately become part of your daily routine.

It generally takes approximately 21 days to form a new habit and 90 days to turn that habit into a permanent lifestyle change. The key is to start implementing new behaviors for a minimum of 21 days and to practice them for at least 90 days until they become a lasting, positive change.

Steps for changing a habit include:
- Becoming aware of the habit and its effect,
- Being self-motivated to change the habit,
- Willingness to take action to change the habit,
- Identifying new habits to put in their place, and

- Taking action by practicing new habits.

STOP is a method that slows down the action so that you can step back and gain more clarity about the link between your thoughts, feelings and the behavior you want to change. the steps include:

- Step outside of yourself.
- Trace your current action back to the motivator.
- Observe your thoughts and clarify your actions.
- Put a new behavior in place of the old behavior.

Three coaching tips to help you gain clarity and begin to implement new habits:

- **Acknowledge Your Feelings**. When you feel hungry, angry, lonely, or tired, recognizing your physical or emotional state is the first step toward managing your feelings effectively.
- **Write in a Journal**. Expressing your feelings in writing can be a therapeutic outlet for exploring your feelings without fear of judgment or confrontation.
- **Seek Support**. If you feel stuck or the situation(s) you face are too much to handle alone, talk to a trusted friend or therapist who can offer perspective, validation, and guidance.

Practice adopting new habits for each of the Motivator categories below

- Busy Lifestyles and Need for Convenience
- Sabotaging Learned Behaviors and Habits
- Life Situations
- HALT (Hungry, Angry, Lonely, Tired)
- Emotional Eating

Emotional eating becomes a problem when this coping mechanism becomes overused and an individual consistently turns to trigger foods for comfort. In contrast to a person who is eating in response to a current, temporary stressor, emotional eaters eat to self-medicate and to numb unwanted feelings, usually those of anxiety, anger, fear or depression, and very often they are reacting to current situations through the lens of past, unresolved trauma

The most common factors that impact stress and emotional eating include:

- Chronic Stress
- Learned Behaviors
- Life Situations/Emotions
- Unresolved Trauma

To Manage Daily Thoughts that Impact Your Habits and Behaviors

- Get support from a coach, therapist, group or individuals such as family or friends if you still find yourself overwhelmed with feelings leading to emotional eating.
- Use a Daily Journal to Document Your Feelings, Stay on Track, and Take Action
- Clean and Organize Your Environment
- Exercise and Spend Time in Nature
- Celebrate Your Accomplishments
- Focus on Progress and Growth
- Acknowledge Your Feelings
- Use a Worry Jar to Release Worries
- Forgive Yourself and Others
- Meditate,
- Practice Deep Breathing
- Identify and Release Anger in a safe way
- Learn to Silence Your Inner Critic
- Surround Yourself with Positive People

Practicing a habit over and over until it becomes automatic is how the brain builds new synaptic connections

A habit tracker is a visual tool that works by providing an easy way to track your progress and stay motivated while you are waiting for the long-term rewards of your efforts to accumulate

The benefits of using a habit tracker in addition to a daily journal include:

- Creating a daily visual set of cues that remind you to act.
- Providing immediate feedback that shows you are on the right path

- Providing encouragement to stick with the habit and achieve consistency
- Helping to improve clarity and insight into your patterns and behavior,
- Providing both motivation and accountability to stay on track

CHAPTER 17
Eliminate Clutter in Your Space to Create an Environment that Supports Lasting Change

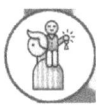

Coach on Your Shoulder

Most books about going sugar-free do not include a chapter on decluttering your home. The connection between quitting sugar and creating an environment free of clutter is not immediately apparent. However, clutter in your physical environment can significantly impact your mental health and ability to make lasting lifestyle changes. While a big part of going sugar-free needs to focus on food plans and success habits (such as getting enough sleep, eating more mindfully, and staying active), equally important is learning how to create a space that supports your ability to focus on changing sabotaging habits and eliminating trigger foods.

A disorganized space often leads to feelings of overwhelm, stress, and mental fatigue, making it harder to stay on track, prepare meals, get restful sleep, and resist impulsive behaviors like reaching for sugary snacks. On the other hand, clearing clutter can create a sense of control and calm, making it easier to reverse old patterns and more consistently implement new behaviors that help you to achieve your goals.

This chapter will explore how to create chaos-free spaces throughout your home that set the stage for mindful living and support your vision of sugar-free, vibrant health. In the context of breaking free from sugar, we will focus on three key areas that impact your ability to make sustainable daily food choices, including your Kitchen, Dining Room, and Bedroom.

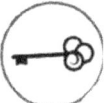

Key Concepts

Addressing Clutter Throughout Your Home in the Context of Creating a Sugar-Free Lifestyle

The Oxford Dictionary defines clutter as "a crowded and untidy collection of things. However, clutter is not about being "messy" or "lazy" or "disorganized." The essence of clutter is surrounding yourself with things you no longer use or love that do not support your physical, mental, and spiritual well-being.

The old saying "your home is your castle" takes on a special meaning when you're trying to break free from sugar and improve your health. The state of your living environment is intertwined with your mental, physical, and spiritual well-being, and your home is a reflection of your inner self. While you can't control the outside world, you can create a safe and supportive environment where your surroundings empower you to feel focused, energized, and calm so that you can achieve your goals.

I experienced this connection during a time when my eating was out of control, and coincidentally, my house was a chaotic mess. I mentioned this to my therapist, who suggested I take a decluttering class offered at my local high school. What an eye-opener! I was fortunate that our teacher had incredible insight into the relationship between the energy in our home and the underlying feelings and behaviors that trigger emotional eating.

Slowly, I began to see how my clutter habits affected my food and eating habits.

Break Free From The Sugar Blues — Janet Sanders

The cookbooks, kitchen tools, gadgets, spices, and other paraphernalia that covered my countertops left me with no space to prepare and cook sugar-free meals, leading to frustration and lots of take-out.

The pantry, full of outdated and disorganized food, had me shopping for things I didn't need, and it also caused me anxiety when I realized I didn't have everything needed to prepare the dish I had planned for dinner. Once I got it all together, I was a pretty good cook, but the entire process was mentally exhausting.

In addition to the general disorder in my kitchen, my crowded refrigerator and freezer made it hard to find anything when I needed it, and I would find myself screaming at it, which made my kids think I was a little bit crazy.

I often wanted to eat in my dining room, but my dining room table, covered with books, mail, magazines, and dishes that didn't fit into my cabinets, left little room for serving a beautiful meal to family or friends. Clearing the table before dinner or entertaining was always a last-minute chore, draining my energy and leaving me feeling cranky and defeated.

My messy bedroom with clothes thrown over chairs, crowded closets, an unmade bed, and work papers piled on my dresser created a chaotic sleeping environment that fed my anxiety and inability to fall asleep.

Living this way was unsustainable, and slowly, I began to address both the inner and outer chaos. When I combined the tools and techniques for eliminating trigger foods and sugar with creating a space that nurtured and supported my sugar-free lifestyle, amazing things started to happen.

I learned that getting rid of clutter was not about letting go of things that were meaningful to me, but rather was focused on letting go of the things that no longer contributed to my life and well-being. By creating a home without all the chaos, I found peace of mind and the energy to focus on building a life I loved. The fun part came when I started to redesign each room, especially my kitchen, which involved filling it with foods that led to new adventures in cooking and nourishing my body in truly transformative ways.

In the remainder of this chapter, we will explore techniques and action steps you can use to keep physical clutter at bay. The purpose is not to impose a minimalist philosophy or force you to eliminate all your stuff. My goal is to share ideas that will help you look at your food life from another perspective so that you can discover ways in which your physical environment is sabotaging your efforts to go sugar-free.

I will begin by teaching you some basic de-cluttering techniques that can be applied to any room in your home. Then, we will focus on the rooms that impact food, eating, and sleeping habits, including your kitchen/pantry, dining areas, and bedroom. In addition to discovering how to de-clutter these spaces, you will learn how to makeover your kitchen and pantry to include the foods and tools that support your sugar-free journey.

Decluttering Basics: Reclaiming Your Space in 4 Steps

The decluttering process combines eliminating things that no longer serve you with creating a space that supports your lifestyle and nurtures your well-being. The basic flow that enables you to transform any space includes observing, sorting, organizing, and enhancing. These decluttering steps are described below.

ANALYZE THE SPACE: Begin by assessing a room to gain clarity about its current state. Observe what's there, how items in the room are being used, and what's not working. Ask yourself:

- What is the function of this space?
- What items genuinely belong here
- What items feel out of place or unnecessary?
- Are there items that constantly create clutter?

SORT & DECIDE WHAT STAYS AND WHAT GOES. This phase is often called sorting your belongings and making mindful decisions about keeping or discarding items that no longer serve you. Things that are no longer useful, broken, redundant, or emotionally draining can be donated, recycled, sold, or discarded. For each item, use the criteria below to decide what stays.

- Is the item useful or necessary? (Does it serve an important function? Do I regularly use it or rely on it?)
- Do I love this item? (It brings genuine happiness having it in my home.)
- Does this item improve my life?

For many, this is the most challenging part of the decluttering process. One person's clutter can be another's prized possession. For example, I love cookbooks. I have hundreds of them. Some people would say, keep a few; the rest are unnecessary. But I use them all the time, and I get joy just looking at them on the shelves and cuddling up on my sofa with a cup of tea to browse through one or two at the end of the day. My dilemma was figuring out how to store them all in a small space. I went through them all and rehomed many before finding shelves that could hold the remainder. Other items that are hard to part with are those with sentimental value. What I ask myself is whether I am keeping a family heirloom or memory out of guilt or whether I truly like having it around. If the latter, I try to find a creative way to keep it in a way that works with the space I have available.

ORGANIZE WHAT YOU KEEP. Once you've pared down your belongings, the next step is to organize what remains. Group similar items together and store them logically. Use containers, shelves, bins, or labels to create order. Make it easy to find what you need and just as easy to put things away. Everything should have a designated place to simplify daily routines.

ENHANCE YOUR SPACE. Finally, think about what would make your newly decluttered space more enjoyable or functional:

- Include items that make it functional based on what you do in the space.
- Boost your mood with items such as plants, pictures, or artwork.
- Improve lighting or add other design elements to make the space inviting
- Ensure the space reflects your personal style and comforts you.

Now that you are familiar with basic decluttering concepts, you are ready to tackle specific rooms, including your kitchen/pantry, dining room (or other eating space), and bedroom. The process for these rooms expands upon the general decluttering concepts with a more detailed focus on creating spaces that support quitting sugar, eliminating trigger foods, and achieving your vision of health.

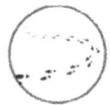

Action Steps

KITCHEN/PANTRY

Decluttering and reorganizing your kitchen and pantry enable you to create a supportive space that empowers easier meal and snack preparation, healthier food choices, and the ability to avoid trigger foods. Before you get into the details of decluttering your kitchen and pantry, take a 3000-foot overview of this space. How do you feel when you enter your kitchen? Do you feel inspired to cook a meal, or do you feel overwhelmed? Are your counter tops and cabinets cluttered? Can you easily find what you need, or are you always searching for things? Do you have food items with added sugar in your refrigerator, freezer, or pantry? What do you like most about your kitchen?

Analyze the Kitchen Space and Sort Items

For efficiency, I combined the first two steps, analyzing and sorting, because, as a practical matter, when decluttering your kitchen, it makes sense to do them together. The first step is taking stock of what you currently have in your kitchen and then deciding what to keep and what to discard from your cabinets, pantry shelves, refrigerator, and freezer. There are several categories of kitchen items that you will be assessing, including food, kitchen tools, appliances, furniture, and storage.

Food

- Go through your pantry shelves, refrigerator, and freezer to read labels and identify foods with added sugar, natural sugar, and hidden sugar. Then determine which food items you want to eliminate, replace with a sugar-free alternative, or store differently. Be aware of items that are trigger foods, and plan to eliminate them. (If consumed by others in your household, store them separately.)

- Spices, Oils & Condiments: Check for stale spices and seasonings, rancid oils, old vinegars, sauces, salad dressings, marinades, and condiments past their best-by or use-by dates.
- Canned and boxed goods: Check for opened items and foods past their best-by or use-by dates
- Refrigerated and frozen items: Check for old/stale refrigerated or frozen items and items in the freezer with freezer burn.

Kitchen Tools and Appliances

- Small tools (such as knives, serving utensils, can openers, whisks, hand-held mandolins, cutting boards, and measuring cups/spoons): Look for duplicates, rusted or broken items, and tools you no longer use. Determine which tools/appliances you will discard or keep, and whether you are missing any that could make meal preparation easier.
- Kitchen furniture and storage, including cabinets, work surfaces, refrigerator/freezer, tables, chairs, trash cans, and other storage.
- Are your cabinets full of dishes, containers, food, or seasonings you never use? Do you have broken dishes or stale food? Identify what you will keep and discard items that you do not need.
- Is there old food lurking in your fridge/freezer? Clean out your refrigerator and freezer, including old items past their use-by or best-by dates.
    - White Potatoes (white potatoes, behave more like simple sugars, breaking down quickly into glucose and causing a sharp insulin response)
    - High sodium processed foods, including high sodium canned foods and meat products
- *Below are some additional ideas for cleaning out your pantry*
    - You don't need to eliminate all foods with saturated fats. However, you should be mindful and carefully consider both the source and the amount.
    - Be careful with fructose in any form. (Eliminate high glycemic fruits, such as raisins)
    - Avoid products containing nitrates

Organize What You Keep

- Categorize your pantry items and group them by type, such as nuts and seeds, condiments, canned goods, spices, and oils. Do the same in your refrigerator so that you can easily find refrigerated items.
- Invest in Clear Containers: Using clear, airtight containers for dry goods such as, quinoa, nuts, seeds, and legumes visually reminds you of your healthy options and simplifies pantry inventory management.
- Organize your spices prominently to encourage experimentation with flavorful dishes that satisfy cravings without sugar.
- Commit to routinely revisiting your pantry. Regularly remove items that have gone stale or that no longer align with your sugar-free goals. This ongoing practice helps sustain your new dietary habits over the long term.

Enhance Your Kitchen Space

Now it is time to have fun by experimenting with new sugar-free alternatives and taking time to explore new ideas that would make your kitchen more enjoyable or functional:

- Research alternatives to foods with added sugar and make replacements as needed. (Refer back to the Action Steps in Chapter 9 for more information about substitutions for food items containing added sugar, natural sugar, and hidden sugar)
- Investigate the purchase of appliances that would make your cooking life easier. (For ideas, refer back to the list of useful kitchen tools outlined in Chapter 16)
- Enhance the space with items such as shelves for cookbooks, plants, pictures, or artwork.
- Improve lighting or add other design elements to make the space inviting. If your kitchen is a gathering place for family and friends, include any storage that will help to keep things in order and clutter at bay.

DINING ROOM AND OTHER EATING AREAS

The state of your dining room, kitchen table or other areas designed for eating such as kitchen islands with stools for seating, can significantly influence eating habits.

Dining room and kitchen tables frequently become dumping grounds for mail, homework, and items that don't fit into kitchen cabinets. It's often easier to avoid this mess rather than clear the table off for meals, leading to chaotic eating habits, that often includes mindless eating in front of the television. It is fine to enjoy movie night with a meal in front of the TV occasionally, and if a space is very small, eating in the living room may not be avoidable. The key is how you feel when you eat in whatever space you choose, and whether you are able to eat in a way that does not encourage overeating or eating trigger foods.

Analyze Dining Spaces

Take a moment to assess your dining room and any other eating areas. Notice what occupies the table, chairs, and any shelves or surfaces. Identify areas that accumulate clutter, making it difficult to enjoy meals comfortably and mindfully.

Some questions to ask as you assess your eating space(s) include:

- How do you feel when you view your dining area(s)?
- Is the table or countertop in your dining area covered with items that must be cleared before you can set the table?
- Do you use the back of chairs to hang coats or other clothing items?
- What types of things are in the dining area that are not needed for eating or serving food?

Sort and Determine What Stays

Evaluate each item and decide what truly belongs in the dining area. Keep only items you genuinely love, frequently use, or that contribute positively to your dining experience. Relocate or donate things that do not fit these criteria.

Remove unnecessary items from the dining table and surrounding areas. Clearing away papers, electronics, and unrelated objects can immediately reduce stress and distraction, creating a peaceful setting for eating

Organize and Enhance the Space: Arrange the remaining items thoughtfully, prioritizing ease of use and visual appeal. Consider adding elements that enhance the dining atmosphere, such as fresh flowers, candles, or attractive table linens, to make the space more enjoyable for regular meals and special celebrations.

THE BEDROOM

Analyze Your Space for Sleeping

Is your sleeping area cluttered, full of electronic equipment, clothes on the back of chairs, or other distractions? Identify areas that accumulate clutter, making it difficult to get sufficient restful sleep.

Some questions to ask as you assess your bedroom include:

- Do you feel relaxed in your bedroom?
- Is your bedroom full of electronic equipment or other distractions?
- Do you have a supportive pillow and mattress?
- Is the lighting conducive to rest and relaxation?
- Do you have enough storage for your clothes, shoes, and other accessories?
- Do you have a nightstand or other furniture next to your bed with space for items such as books, reading glasses, water bottles, or medications?

Sort and Determine What Stays

Evaluate each item and decide what truly belongs in your bedroom. Keep only items you genuinely love, frequently use, or that contribute to restful sleep. Relocate or donate things that do not fit these criteria.

If you currently use your bedroom as an office, rethink this arrangement. Make your bedroom a place to rest, not a room where you are reminded of stressful situations. Clearing away dirty clothes, papers, electronics, and unrelated objects can immediately create a peaceful setting for sleeping.

Organize and Enhance the Space:

If you have a television or tablet for reading in the bedroom, get in the habit of turning them off at least 30 minutes before you fall asleep. If you need to have your

Takeaways & Highlights

The four steps for de-cluttering include: Analyzing, Sorting, Organizing and Enhancing the space.

Decluttering your kitchen/pantry involves the reorganization of three main categories of items, including the following.

- Food in your cabinets, pantry, refrigerator and freezer
- Kitchen tools and small appliances
- Kitchen furniture and storage such as cabinets, work surfaces, refrigerator/freezer, tables, chairs, trash cans, and other storage

Analyzing your food items requires reading labels. How to read labels to find sugar was discussed in Chapter 9. Below is a summary of tips for reading and understanding food labels.

- Food labels have a Nutrition Facts and an Ingredients section, which provide different types of information. Ingredients are listed in order, starting with the ingredient found in the largest amount, by weight, and progressing to the ingredient present in the smallest amount
- The FDA definition of "sugar," as found in the Code of Federal Regulations, means the natural sweet substance "obtained from sugar cane or sugar beets." The term "sugars" on a nutrition label means the sum of different types of sugars (such as glucose, fructose, lactose, and sucrose).
- The Nutrition Label contains a separate section for all sugars and for added sugar. The amount of total sugar grams equals the sum of added Sugars plus natural sugars.

- Added sugar means any sugar that is added during processing or as part of food preparation.
- Natural sugar means sugars that are found naturally in foods, such as lactose in dairy products, fructose in fruit, and maltose, which is found in a variety of foods, including grains.
- A food that claims to have no added sugar means that NO sugar or ingredient containing sugar was added during processing or packaging, but it may still contain some natural sugar or artificial sweeteners.
- A food that claims it is Sugar-Free (a.k.a. zero sugar, sugarless) means that One Serving contains less than 0.5 grams of sugar (it might contain natural or added sugar).
- Total Carbohydrate: This reflects the total amount of carbohydrates in the food product. In the nutrition facts table, the number of total carbohydrates means the sum of sugar, starches, and dietary fiber. Although all sugars are classified as carbohydrates, not all carbohydrates are sugars.

Janet's Pantry

People often ask me what my "must-have" kitchen and pantry items are. Here is a list of the food items I always keep on hand. We all have different tastes and priorities, and your needs may be different than mine. Use this list as a starting point, taking into consideration your specific needs, food plan, and trigger foods.

- **Non-Starchy Vegetables**
- **Yams/Sweet Potatoes**
- **Frozen Peas, Frozen Corn (Fresh Corn in Season)**
- **Other Vegetables**
    - Carrots
    - Cauliflower (Fresh, Frozen Florets, and Riced)
    - Cucumbers
    - Frozen Edamame
    - Fresh & Minced Garlic, Fresh Ginger
    - Green & Red Cabbage
    - Kale, Celery, Iceberg, and Romaine Lettuce
    - Onions, Tomatoes

- o Peppers (red, yellow, green)
- o Mushrooms (fresh and dried)
- **Fruit**
  - o Acai Berry (Powder & Frozen)
  - o Blueberries (Frozen & Fresh in summer)
  - o Citrus Fruits (Lemons, Limes)
- **Whole Grains**
  - o Barley
  - o Quinoa (Red & White)
  - o Steel Cut Oats
- **Nuts, Seeds & Nut Butters**
  - o Almonds, Pecans, Walnuts
  - o Raw Pumpkin Seeds
  - o Roasted Sunflower Seeds
  - o Ground Flax Seeds & Chia Seeds
  - o Almond Butter, Peanut Butter
  - o Tahini
- **Beans**
  - o Canned: Garbanzo, Black, Navy, Mixed Beans for Salad/Chili
  - o Dried: Lentils, Adzuki Beans
  - o Hummus & Other Bean Spreads
- **Marinades & Stir Fry Seasonings**
  - o No sugar added Marinades
  - o Bragg's Liquid Amino Acids
  - o Ponzu Sauce (no sugar added)
  - o Tamari
- **Healthy Fats & Oils**
  - o Olive Oil (Extra Virgin)
  - o Avocados
  - o Other Oils: Coconut, Walnut, Avocado
- **Seasonings**
  - o Cinnamon, Vanilla, Turmeric, Pepper, Cilantro, Chili Powder, Paprika, Parsley, Garam Masala, Gomashio, Sea Salt, Trader Joe's 21 Salute
- **Bread, Wraps, Crackers & Baking Products**

- Sprouted Grain Bread, English Muffins,
- Keto/Low Carb Bread, Wraps & Tortillas
- Alternative flours: Almond, Coconut
- Baking Soda, Baking Powder
- Keto Pancake Mix

- **Vinegar, Salad Dressings, Marinades**
  - Vinegar: Red Wine, Balsamic, Rice, Ume Plum, Citrus Flavored, Apple Cider
  - No Added Sugar Salad Dressings

- **Dairy, Protein & Milk Alternatives**
  - Fish, Grass Fed Beef, Organic Poultry
  - Goat Cheese (spreadable & regular)
  - Plain Yogurt (Greek, Skyr)
  - Cottage Cheese
  - Cheese (cubed, sliced, shredded)
- Fresh Parmesan Cheese
  - Part Skim Ricotta
  - Tofu (Firm & Silky)
  - Butter (Grass Fed)
  - Unsweetened Almond Milk
  - Lite Coconut Milk
  - Sardines
  - Pasture Raised, Organic Eggs

- **Condiments, & Miscellaneous**
  - Mustard
  - Mayonnaise (No Sugar Added)
  - Sun Dried Tomatoes,
  - Marinated Artichoke Hearts
  - Capers
  - Greens Powder, Whey Protein Powder
  - Soup Stock (Vegetable/Chicken)
  - Bone Broth
  - Worcestershire Sauce,
  - Salsa
  - Unsweetened Raw Cacao
  - Goji Powder

- Dark Chocolate (70%, Sugar-free)
- Tea (Decaffeinated Green & Black)
- Seltzer & Sparkling Water
- Tomato Sauce/Pasta Sauce/Pizza Sauce
- Stevia, Monk Fruit, Allulose (Powder and Liquid)
- Toasted Nori Sheets (large for sushi and small for snacking)

CHAPTER 18
Enjoy Life

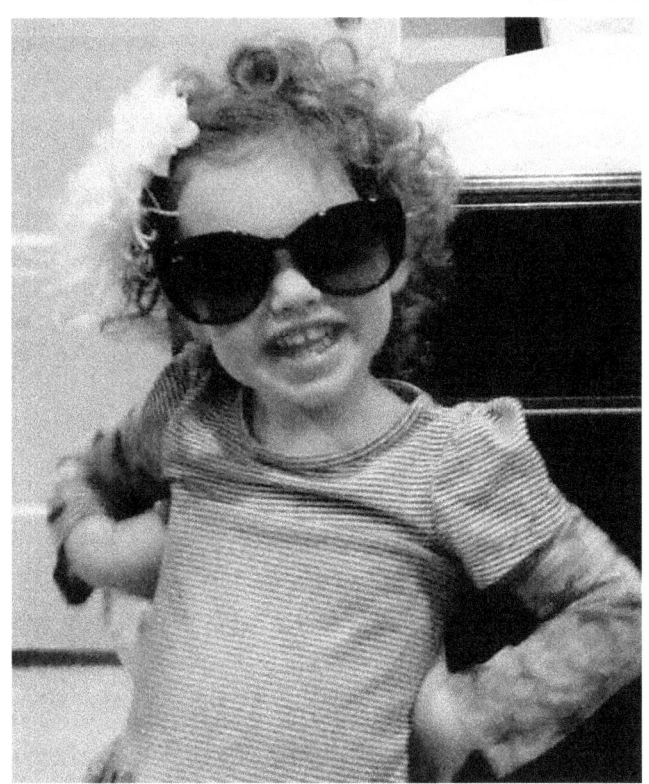

Coach on Your Shoulder

It is a real art to learn how to create and maintain a sugar-free lifestyle without letting it overtake all of your thoughts and energy. Getting through each day without constantly thinking about what to eat and how to avoid trigger foods is where success habits and learning to manage your mind come in.

Taking care of yourself in a new way is challenging. Whether you choose to drain your mental energy by thinking negatively about changing your lifestyle is totally within your control. When you find it difficult to feel positively about doing "one more thing" to stay sugar-free and to manage emotional or stress eating, take a minute to recall your vision of health and the goals you hope to achieve.

It may be hard to imagine now, but you will find that practicing success habits that support your ability to avoid trigger foods that can lead to physical addiction to sugar are a reward unto themselves. It's a self-perpetuating cycle. The better you start to feel, the more you want to do the things that move you towards your vision and help you feel better.

Remember, habits are repeated behaviors that ultimately become automatic. In the beginning, you put a lot of time and effort into things like remembering to eat certain foods, to drink more water, to plan meals, and to fit in exercise. But, over time, they will become part of your routine, and your mind will dwell less on the negative and shift to your overall well-being.

You will incorporate success habits such as taking a morning walk, asking the waiter not to bring bread to the table, skipping the sugary desserts, keeping a bottle of water with you, and avoiding trigger foods, all without the relentless voice in your head going on and on about what you are missing.

Life is short. Creating and maintaining a sugar-free lifestyle is not about deprivation. To the contrary, you will take care of yourself better than you ever have. Dare to believe that you are going to enjoy yourself and live life to the fullest. What could be better?

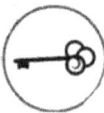

Key Concepts

Make Your Well-Being a Priority

Making sustainable changes means creating a balanced approach where pleasure and well-being coexist. Many people mistakenly perceive self-care as selfishness. However, taking care of yourself ensures you have the energy, clarity, and resilience to face challenges and make difficult choices. Investing in your health at all levels is an act of self-respect, enabling you to show up as your best self for yourself, family, friends, and your community.

Putting yourself first and prioritizing your health when adopting a sugar-free lifestyle is essential for long-term success. Here are steps you can take to maintain enjoyment and overall wellness during your lifestyle transformation:

- Practice mindfulness by savoring meals and appreciating new flavors, fostering joy in eating rather than restriction.
- Engage in hobbies and creative activities to stimulate your mind, reduce stress, and cultivate personal satisfaction beyond dietary changes.
- Connect socially by nurturing meaningful relationships with family and friends, which enriches emotional health and provides support.
- Prioritize rest and self-care through adequate sleep, relaxation techniques, and personal rituals that restore your energy and spirit.
- Celebrate your successes and milestones, reinforcing positive feelings toward your new lifestyle and enhancing self-confidence.

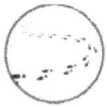

Action Steps

Little Luxuries to Enjoy Life While Going Sugar Free

Remember to have fun and incorporate little luxuries into your day. Here are some ideas.

- **Wake up early, sip a hot beverage** (bone broth, tea, morning coffee), and spend some quiet time meditating or writing in your journal.
- **Light scented candles or essential oils** to create a relaxing atmosphere.
- **Take a leisurely walk or hike in nature**. Experience the colors and sounds of nature and connect with your surroundings.
- **Have lunch with a friend**. Enjoy good conversation and fine food.

- **Cook up a perfect pot of chili or favorite casserole**. Set your table with festive plates and flowers, and invite some friends to share a meal.
- **Practice gentle yoga or stretching routines** to reconnect with your body. Uncontrolled stress raises cortisol levels and can affect food choices, blood sugars, and weight. Yoga is just one of many great ways to de-stress.
- **Spend an afternoon with a good book** or chill out with a few of your favorite magazines.
- **Enjoy a warm cup of tea in a beautiful cup**. Try teas from different countries: Earl Grey/English Breakfast (England), Darjeeling (India), Matcha/Kukicha (Japan), Jasmine/White Tea (China), Rooibos (South Africa), Ceylon Tea (Sri Lanka), Lemon Balm/Lemon Verbena (Greece)
- **Concoct a magnificent sugar-free afternoon high tea** and share it with friends or family.
- **Go dancing**. It is a great way to have fun and get extra exercise.
- **Create a relaxing playlist** of soothing or inspiring music.
- **Book a massage or spa treatment** to unwind and celebrate reaching health milestones.
- **Try a new hobby or class**—something you've always wanted to learn.
- **Treat yourself to fresh flowers** to brighten your living space
- **Take a relaxing bubble bath or long shower** to soothe and pamper yourself
- **Spend time with a furry friend**. Walking a dog not only provides physical exercise but also serves as a time for reflection, promoting mental clarity and emotional stability. A cat's soothing purr and gentle presence have been shown to positively affect mental, emotional, and even physical well-being.
- **Visit local parks, museums, or galleries** to nourish your creativity.
- **Buy yourself a cozy blanket or comfortable pajamas** to enhance relaxation time.
- **Go to a movie, or have a movie night at home**.
- **Browse through a bookstore**. Treat yourself to a new cookbook and experiment with new recipes or ingredients.
- **Keep a gratitude journal**. Reflect daily on things you're thankful for.
- **Take a personal day and do whatever comes to mind**. Let the day take you wherever it leads, and let your mind run free.

Takeaways & Highlights

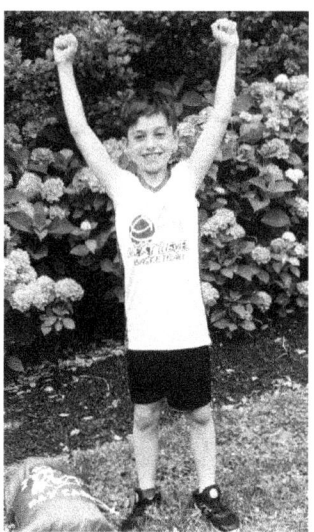

COMING FULL CIRCLE:
The 4 C's of Change and Resilience

Congratulations on completing the steps in the Sugar-Free Lifestyle Roadmap™. As you continue on your sugar-free journey, keep the 4 C's of change and resilience close and use them every day to move forward towards a life you love.

COMMIT to your goals and future vision.
CONNECT with yourself and a nurturing community of support.
Practice CONSISTENCY, and never give up.
Let mental and physical CLARITY be your daily guide.
Always remember that yesterday holds your memories,
and tomorrow chases your dreams.
Only today gives you the chance to connect with yourself,
to enjoy your life, and change the way you walk through this world.

APPENDIX A
Coach & Cook Guide

How Improvisational Cooking Can Help You Create Satisfying Meals and Snacks

A key to my success in changing my relationship with sugar was learning to be creative in the kitchen and finding ways to prepare sugar-free foods that meet my needs. We all have different food preferences, and trying to stay on someone else's food plan can be a recipe for disaster. Cooking for myself and my family based on the things we enjoy eating was a gift that transformed my health and is one of the foundations of my sugar-free lifestyle. Although I am a big fan of cookbooks (I have over 100 in my collection), I discovered that learning how to use recipes as a guide and inspiration for dishes that were easy to prepare, while being more creative in the kitchen, was a big part of not getting bored and staying away from trigger foods.

Today, when it comes to day-to-day cooking, I most often employ a free-form approach, often referred to as improvisational cooking. It is a fluid type of food preparation that will enable you to prepare satisfying and delicious meals more spontaneously with what you have on hand. One of the cookbooks I used for guidance when starting this new way of cooking was "How to Cook Without a Book" by Pam Anderson. I have listed some other cookbooks and recipe sources in the Suggested Reading and Resources section.

The common denominator for this type of food preparation is the idea that recipes serve as guides based on a formula for a particular type of food or dish. Sometimes I start from scratch without a recipe, and at other times, I use a recipe as a starting point. Once you understand the basic formula underlying a specific recipe or cooking style (such as sauté, stir-fry, roast, braise, etc.), you can swap out ingredients and adjust amounts based on what is available, as well as your own tastes and preferences.

Different chefs use different approaches to improvisational cooking. My Coach & Cook recipes feature both a coaching component, where I explain the ingredients and provide a basic formula for preparing the dish, as well as detailed preparation techniques. The key is to understand basic techniques and how recipes work; then, the possibilities are endless. You can embellish and add from there based on your taste and creativity.

Whether you're using a traditional or free-form recipe, the key is to remain flexible. It is always fine to swap out ingredients or adjust the amount of an ingredient based on taste and the number of people you are preparing food for. (The one exception is baking, where measurements generally should be followed for optimum results)

For example, if you are using a recipe for a stir fry that calls for string beans and you don't have any, substitute broccoli. If you find a great smoothie recipe that includes peanut butter and you only have almond butter on hand, use that instead. Don't want to thicken your smoothie with sugar-laden bananas? I have a smoothie for breakfast every day, and I haven't had a banana in years. If I find a recipe with a banana that looks good, I substitute ice for the thickener and stevia for sweetness. Have a great French Toast recipe? Swap out the grain-based flour bread and use a Paleo or sprouted grain bread instead.

If you're unsure how much of an ingredient or seasoning to add, the best technique is to add a little at a time. A little common sense comes in handy here. I very often do a taste test as I go along. However, not if I am preparing raw foods. I might taste a spoonful of mashed sweet potatoes to see if I have added enough cinnamon, and I might taste a marinade BEFORE pouring it over raw chicken. However, I will not taste ingredients poured over raw poultry until the chicken has been thoroughly cooked. At the end, before serving, I might taste to see if anything extra is needed.

In this appendix, I have included a few basic Coach & Cook recipes to help you get started and provide some ideas for dishes that I have found to be foundations for a sugar-free lifestyle.

Breakfast Ideas

<u>Yogurt Parfait</u>

Parfaits are great for a quick breakfast, as a snack, or served as an elegant dessert. You can also substitute cottage cheese for the yogurt. The key is to use plain yogurt without added sugar and to limit the amount and type of fruit you use.

Basic Preparation: Yogurt + Protein Powder + Sweetener of Choice + Flavoring of Choice] + Layered Low Glycemic Fruit + Garnish/Crunch

INGREDIENTS:

- Plain Yogurt: One cup of yogurt will yield 2 small parfaits. Greek or Icelandic (Skyr) Yogurt are both creamy and low in natural sugar.
- Sweetener of Choice (to taste)
- 1/2-1 tsp Protein Powder: Gives the yogurt a pudding consistency and adds more protein. (optional)
- Flavoring(s): I use cinnamon and a touch of vanilla to flavor the yogurt. If you enjoy chocolate, consider adding some unsweetened cocoa powder. You could also use a flavored Liquid Stevia.
- Fruit of choice (Suggested: fresh or frozen blueberries, raspberries, and/or strawberries. (Approx. a cup of fruit for two parfaits.) Choose low-glycemic fruits, such as berries, and avoid high-glycemic fruits, including melons, grapes, and ripe bananas.
- "Crunch": I make "crunch" using Ezekiel 4:9 Almond Sprouted Whole Grain Cereal. (See Instructions). In place of crunch, you can substitute chopped walnuts, pecans, or a grain-free granola.

INSTRUCTIONS:

Prepare the Crunch: Heat up a heavy skillet, and add 1/4 to 1/2 box of Ezekiel 4:9 Almond Sprouted Whole Grain Cereal to the skillet. Sprinkle some cinnamon over the cereal, and then sprinkle dry sweetener of choice (or pour a small amount of liquid sweetener such as sugar-free maple syrup) over the cereal.

Next, mix the cinnamon and sweetener into the cereal, stirring it for about 5 minutes over low heat to slightly roast the cereal mixture. Remove from the heat and put in a bowl to cool. Depending on the sweetener used, the mixture may stick together when it cools down. Use a fork to break it apart gently.

Prepare the Yogurt and Fruit: Place the yogurt in a bowl and add the Protein Powder. Then add a small amount of sweetener and a pinch of cinnamon. Mix the sweetener and cinnamon into the yogurt. Taste, and add more sweetener and cinnamon if needed. Wash & rinse the fruit. If using strawberries, cut them into small pieces

Assemble the Parfaits: Place a tablespoon of the crunch in the bottom of the glasses or parfait glasses. Next, place approximately 1/4 cup of the yogurt on top of the crunch. Top with 1/4 cup of the fruit. Repeat the layers.

Egg Muffins

These egg muffins are versatile, making it easy to customize them with your favorite vegetables, cheese, or protein. You can bake them in the oven or use an electric appliance to prepare "egg bites".

Basic Preparation: Sauteed Vegetables + Eggs + Spices + Optional Protein + Pour Ingredients into Muffin Containers & Bake (Or Use Appliance to Create Egg Bites)

SUGGESTED INGREDIENTS FOR VEGGIE EGG MUFFINS

- 8-12 Eggs (enough for 12 muffin cups – amount may vary based on size of eggs and amount of vegetables, cheese or protein added)
- 1 cup red pepper, chopped
- 1 cup mushrooms, sliced
- 4 cups spinach (chopped into small pieces, or use baby leaf spinach) [substitute chopped broccoli if you are not a fan of spinach].
- ½ tsp garlic powder
- Dash of pepper
- Optional (1/2 tsp turmeric).

INSTRUCTIONS:

Preheat your oven to 350°F. Place 12 muffin cups in muffin tin (or you can lightly grease or spray a NONSTICK muffin tray with a light coating of oil of choice.) If you're going to line them, be sure to get good quality non-stick liners --the same texture as parchment or baking paper).

Sauté pepper and mushrooms for about 3 minutes until crisp-tender. Add spinach and cook until wilted.

In a separate bowl, whisk eggs and spices together until blended

Combine egg mixture with sautéed vegetables and then pour into 12 muffin cups. It's ok if they only fill halfway because these will expand in the oven.

Place in oven and bake about 15-20 minutes, (or until eggs have set). (Optionally, you can use an electric appliance to make egg bites instead of muffins.)

Breakfast Chaffles

All you need is a Mini or Regular Size Waffle maker. Dash makes a mini waffle maker that is reasonably priced. They also make a larger size that makes 4 chaffles at once. The amounts below are for 1-2 chaffles. You can double the recipe for four, etc.).

Basic Preparation: Egg + Cheese of Choice + Flavoring or Sweetener of Choice + [Optional: Small Amount of Non-Grain Based Flour]

INGREDIENTS: [for 1-2 breakfast chaffles]

- 1 large egg
- 1 heaping tablespoon of light cream cheese [You can substitute full-fat if you prefer, but, for best results, do not use no-fat cream cheese. I generally use cream cheese for breakfast chaffles, and cheeses such as grated cheddar or mozzarella for savory chaffles.
- Flavoring or Sweetener of Choice: Add a small amount of flavoring, such as vanilla, and/or sweetener of choice. You can also add a small amount of unsweetened cacao powder for a chocolate chaffle.
- Optional: 1/2 - 1 tsp of non-grain-based flour of choice (this is optional, but I find it improves the texture and makes the final product less "eggy". You can

use almond flour, coconut flour, or a premixed Keto pancake mix, such as BirchBenders.]
- Optional: Toppings such as melted butter, sugar-free syrup, sugar-free honey, sliced fruit, or fruit compote [You can also create savory chaffles to make breakfast sandwiches]

INSTRUCTIONS:

Beat one egg in a bowl until smooth.

Add cream cheese. You can gently mash it along the side of the bowl with a spoon to make it easier to incorporate into the egg with a whisk, until the mixture is well blended. For best results, let cream cheese sit out to soften before adding to the recipe

Add non-grain-based flour and any other seasonings or sweeteners of choice, and whisk until mixture is well blended.

Plug in the chaffle maker and when hot, if desired, place a very small amount of butter in the bottom. (This is optional, I find it helps the chaffle not to stick.)

As soon as the butter melts, pour in the chaffle mix. The secret to preventing the chaffle from overflowing is to pour in an amount that does not overfill the bottom of the chaffle maker. (By doing this, you can also get two chaffles from the ingredients instead of one.

Close the cover and let the chaffle cook. You will see some steam coming out from the sides; that is normal. After about a minute, open the chaffle maker to make sure your chaffle is not burning. Close the lid for 30 seconds to a minute and recheck it.

When done, remove the chaffle and enjoy with toppings or no-sugar syrup of choice.

To make a simple blueberry compote, place blueberries and a small amount of butter in a pan. Heat over low heat, gently mashing the blueberries as they cook. You can add a little water if needed. I also sweeten with a bit of monk fruit. When done, pour over your chaffle.

Cook until the underside of the toast is golden brown and the egg is set on the bottom (about 1-2 minutes). Do not overcook.

Using a spatula, gently turn the bread/egg over and cook until the yolk is cooked to your liking. If you want the yolk to be "runny", only cook for a brief moment and then remove the bread/egg from the skillet with a spatula, turning it back over as you place it on your plate. (If you want the yoke to be less runny, cook it a little longer.)

Sprinkle with salt and pepper to taste.

Super Berry Smoothie

There is no right or wrong way to make a smoothie. With one caveat, avoid ingredients high in sugar and/or fructose. Stick with low-glycemic fruits, such as berries, and limit your intake of bananas. Also, always try to add some protein or fiber. You can add extras for different tastes, health benefits, and textures. If you are using ice as a thickener, use a blender with sufficient power to crush the ice so that it doesn't remain in chunks, resulting in a smooth drink.

Basic Preparation: Liquid + Thickener +Protein/Fiber +Fruit/Vegetables + Sweetener of Choice + Optional Nutrition Boosters and Flavorings

INGREDIENTS:

- ½- 1 cups unsweetened Vanilla Almond Milk (depending on thickness*) (or "milk" of choice)
- 1-2 scoops of Vanilla Protein Powder (Plant-Based or Whey Protein Powder)
- 2 teaspoons almond butter (or nut butter/seed butter of choice)
- ½ cup frozen blueberries (I like to use frozen wild blueberries)
- 1 packet frozen Sugar-Free Acai Berry Puree
- 4-6 Ice cubes (as desired, the more ice cubes, the thicker the smoothie)
- ½ tsp vanilla and/or cinnamon (optional)
- OPTIONAL: 1 tbsp. Goji Powder, Sweetener of Choice

INSTRUCTIONS:

Pour the Almond Milk into a blender

Add the remaining ingredients.

Blend the ingredients until smooth.

Pour into a glass and enjoy!

Ingredients For Green Chocolate Smoothie:

- ½ -1 cup unsweetened Chocolate Almond Milk (or "milk" of Choice)
- 1-2 scoops of Chocolate Protein Powder (Plant-Based or Whey Protein)
- 2 teaspoons of almond butter (or nut butter/seed butter of choice)
- 1 Scoop chocolate flavored Greens Powder
- 1 tbsp. raw Cacao powder
- 4-6 Ice cubes (as desired, the more ice cubes, the thicker the smoothie)
- OPTIONAL: 1 1/2 tablespoons ground flax seed, sweetener of choice

Try adding a small amount of avocado for extra creaminess, additional fiber, and healthy monounsaturated fat, or add a small amount of frozen blueberries for extra sweetness and antioxidants. If you like bananas and are not overly concerned about a small additional amount of natural sugar, add a very small piece of fresh or frozen banana (1/4 to 1/2). Make sure the banana is NOT overly ripe.

Snacks, Sides & Heartier Dishes

Snack Boxes

The possibilities for mix-and-match snack boxes are endless. Assemble 3-4 ingredients from different food groups, and you have a filling snack to look forward to. If you prefer to have one of these boxes as a meal, boost your portion sizes.

PROTEIN	FRUITS
Hardboiled Eggs	Oranges
Hummus/Spreads	Blueberries
Cheese	Raspberries
Jerky	Blackberries
"Nova" Lox or Smoked Salmon	Strawberries
Tuna/Chicken Salad	**VEGGIES**
Uncured Deli Meat	Celery
Chickpeas/Beans	Carrots
Roasted Chicken	Cucumber Slices
	Broccoli Florets
FATS	Bell Peppers
Avocado/Guacamole	Snap Peas
Almonds	Cherry Tomatoes
Walnuts	Artichoke Hearts
Pecans	Roasted Vegetables
Olives	

Quick Cucumber Salads

The easiest way to slice the cucumbers for this salad is to use a handheld mandolin. I own one made by Kyocera, and it is invaluable for preparing vegetables quickly. Be careful as you approach the end of the cucumber or other vegetables. The blade is very sharp. Always use the guard that comes with the mandolin to protect your fingers, or wear a protective glove specially made for use with cutting.

Basic Preparation: Sliced or Diced Cucumber + Vinegar or Citrus (Lemon/Lime) + Flavorings (Salty, Sweet) Optional: Small Amount of Oil of Choice, Dairy Such as Sour Cream for a Creamy Salad

INGREDIENTS:

- Cucumber (I like to use an English Cucumber or 2-3 smaller Kirby Cucumbers)
- Rice Vinegar (or vinegar of choice, such as white balsamic) (to taste, start small -- 1 TBSP, taste and add more if desired)
- Mirin (to taste - start small, 1/2 tsp, taste, then add more if desired)
- Dash of Tamari, Coconut, or Bragg Liquid Aminos (or you could use Ponzu Sauce)

- Optional: sprinkle sesame seeds or the seasoning Gomashio on top of your salad and garnish with sliced carrots or radishes

INSTRUCTIONS:

Slice cucumbers thinly.

Next pour rice vinegar (use a brand without added sugar) over the cucumbers.

Next: season with a little Mirin and/or Bragg Liquid Amino All Purpose Seasoning to taste.

Alternatively, you could season the cucumbers with Ponzu Sauce (an Asian seasoning that is a combination of Rice Vinegar, Mirin and Tamari) (use the liquid sparingly and season to taste)

Basic Cauliflower Rice

Cauliflower rice is made by pulsing cauliflower in a food processor or blender into granules that are roughly the size of rice. Alternatively, the cauliflower can be shredded with a box grater. If you are pressed for time, no need to make your own. Cauliflower rice can be found pre-riced in the produce section of most grocery stores or packaged in the frozen vegetable section. Do not expect the taste and texture to be exactly like white or brown rice. However, the neutral undertones of cauliflower make it very versatile, and it is easy to add different seasonings or vegetables, such as sautéed onions, to transform its taste. It can be served just like rice as a side dish for curry, stir fry, or beans. Alternatively, it can be a dish on its own, such as fried rice, or used as a filling for tacos and burritos. The simplest way to prepare basic cauliflower rice is to sauté it with some olive oil or butter and season it with salt and pepper.

Basic Preparation: Riced Cauliflower + (Optional Lightly Steam + Press Out Liquid) + Sauté + Season + Add Any Sautéed Vegetables or Condiments

INGREDIENTS:

- 1 Head of cauliflower
- 1 TBSP Olive Oil (or oil of choice)

- Seasonings of Choice/To Taste (Bragg Liquid Aminos, Tamari, Salt, Pepper, Gomashio, Red Pepper Flakes, Parsley, Cilantro, Seasoning Mix such as Trader Joe's 21 Salute)

INSTRUCTIONS:

Cut one head of cauliflower in half and cut the florets off from core

Break up the florets into somewhat evenly sized pieces

Place the florets in the bowl of a food processor in batches. Process until evenly chopped but not completely pulverized. (I use a Vitamix for this step using the pulse feature to pulse the contents until they are reduced to the size of couscous or rice grains.) If there are large pieces, remove and process separately. (Be careful, you don't want to "puree" the cauliflower into mush!) Another option is to "rice" the cauliflower using a box grater with medium-sized holes - either way is fine

OPTIONAL: My process is to very slightly pre-cook the cauliflower before sautéing it. This is a preference. If you are in a hurry, you can skip this step. (or maybe try it once to see if you like the results) The idea is NOT to fully cook the cauliflower at this point, but to get it a little bit soft. I have found this helps so that you don't have to under-cook or over-cook it in the "sauté" step of cooking. (you don't want the finished dish to be too crunchy or too "mushy").

To Pre-Cook: Place cauliflower rice in a microwave safe bowl, sprinkle it with a little water and placed a paper towel, paper plate or other microwave safe cover over the bowl. Place the bowl in the microwave for 45 seconds to 1 minute. Remove bowl from microwave and proceed to Step #3. (NOTE: If you do not have a microwave, you can use a steam basket to steam for 1 minute.)

Heat olive oil in a large pan over medium heat

If you have not pre-cooked the cauliflower rice, add it in one layer to the heated oil. Then, place a lid on the pan and let the cauliflower cook for 1-2 minutes. Then, stir and continue cooking for an additional 2-3 minutes. (until tender, not mushy). Then season as desired. (Ideas: salt, pepper, red pepper flakes, seasoning mix, parsley, cilantro)

If you have pre-cooked the cauliflower rice, it is helpful to press out any excess moisture by transferring it to a paper towel or absorbent dish towel and gently squeezing or pressing to remove any remaining water. This ensures no excess moisture remains, which can make your dish soggy. Next, add the cauliflower rice in one layer to the heated oil. There is no need to place a top over the pan. Sauté and stir occasionally for 3-5 minutes, then season to taste.

If desired, garnish with other vegetables, nuts, or sunflower seeds. For a simple meal, I like to add sautéed onions or cooked petite peas.

Let the Salmon Rest. Let it Rest. Remove your salmon from the heat and allow it to rest for 5 minutes. This crucial step ensures several things:

Even Doneness: Heat continues to distribute throughout the fillet, preventing overcooked edges and a raw center.

Juiciness: Resting lets the salmon's juices reabsorb into the flesh, resulting in a succulent, not dry, final product.

Quinoa Many Ways

QUINOA is actually a pseudocereal, meaning it's a seed that cooks like a grain. Since quinoa is botanically considered a seed, it offers more protein than traditional grains (8 grams per cooked cup) and provides a source of complete protein. (Which means that it provides all nine essential amino acids). Thanks to its low glycemic index and high fiber content, quinoa releases energy slowly, which helps to prevent sudden blood glucose spikes and crashes. It is a very versatile grain that is as delicious as a hearty salad, a hot side dish, or when served as a hot cereal for breakfast.

Basic Preparation: Cooked Quinoa + Prepared Vegetables (+ Protein, if desired) +Seasoning + Garnish

Rinse one cup of quinoa thoroughly with cool water in a fine-mesh strainer until the water runs clear. ALWAYS rinse quinoa before cooking to thoroughly remove the bitter coating, called saponin, which is a naturally occurring toxin that coats the quinoa grain. Quinoa is rinsed before packaging to remove the saponin, but it is best to rinse again before cooking.

Combine the quinoa and 2 cups water in a saucepan. Cover and bring to a boil. (for extra flavor you can cook in vegetable or chicken broth)

Reduce the heat to a simmer and continue to cook covered for about 15 minutes or until all the water has been absorbed.

If serving on its own, let the quinoa sit for a few moments, and then plump it up with a fork before placing it in a bowl to serve.

SERVING IDEAS

Emerald Quinoa: Cook Quinoa. While quinoa is cooking, sauté diced onion until soft and sweet tasting. Set onions aside. Lightly boil some kale, and chop it up finely. Lightly boil some Broccoli crowns and cut them into small pieces. Put ¼ cup frozen peas in a strainer and run under very hot water for 3-4 minutes until thawed. Mix the all of the vegetables in with the quinoa. Season with your choice of: Gomashio, Bragg Liquid Aminos, Salt, Ponzu Sauce, or Tamari Soy Sauce. (Use the liquid sparingly and season to taste.)

Quinoa with Peas, Onions and Chopped Arugula: Prepare Quinoa per directions and store in refrigerator. Sauté onion and store in refrigerator. At mealtime: Defrost ½ cup of frozen peas by placing in strainer and running under hot water for 2-3 minutes. Put small amount of olive oil in skillet. Add the quinoa, onions and peas. Sauté lightly for 2-3 minutes. Add chopped arugula. Sauté for another minute. Season to taste. Garnish with Nuts or Seeds of choice. (if desired add some canned beans or leftover fish/chicken).

Quinoa with Sundried Tomatoes, Onions & Corn: Cook Quinoa. While quinoa is cooking, sauté diced onion until soft and sweet tasting. Lightly steam 2 ears of corn and remove corn from the cob. Dice enough sundried tomatoes to measure ¼ cup. Add all ingredients to the Quinoa. Season to taste with an all-purpose seasoning blend such as Trader Joe's 21 Salute, Bragg Liquid Amino Acids, or Tamari Soy Sauce.

Quinoa with Black Bean Salsa: Cook Quinoa. Set aside. Rinse contents of one can of black beans. Mix beans with diced red and orange bell peppers, chopped tomato, and chopped red onion. Drizzle small amount of olive oil over the beans and mix well. Add rice vinegar to taste. If desired, add some chopped cilantro and/or sprinkle with some lime juice. Add bean mixture to the quinoa.

Roasted Sweet Potatoes

I often roast a batch of sweet potatoes on Sunday and use them in a variety of recipes throughout the week, such as Sweet Potato Home Fries with Sautéed Onions and Peppers, a Warm Lentil and Sweet Potato Salad, or a Sweet Potato Stew or Soup that I can prepare in a Crockpot. There are many different types of sweet potatoes, including Jewel, Red Garnet, Japanese, Beauregard, Covington, and Centennial. Often, the terms "sweet potato" and "yam" are used interchangeably, but this can be confusing because true yams are not sweet potatoes, and they are difficult to find at most grocery stores. Sweet potatoes have smoother skin, and their flesh can be white, orange, or even purple. In contrast, true yams have thicker, rougher skin, and their flesh ranges from white to reddish, but it is usually white.

Basic Preparation: Sweet Potatoes Cut into Desired Shape + Oil of Choice + Seasonings [Roast + Add Garnishes, If Desired, Such As Toasted Pecans]

INSTRUCTIONS:

Prepare: You can leave the skins on for added taste and nutrients, or peel the potatoes. Try it both ways and see which you prefer. If you are leaving the skins on, scrub the potatoes thoroughly with a vegetable brush and dry them well before slicing. If you are peeling the potatoes, wash them first.

Cut: On a cutting board, cut off and discard the ends of the potatoes.

Roasted Rounds: Slice the potato into rounds about ¼ inch thick.

Roasted Cubes: First, slice into rounds about ½ inch thick, then slice the rounds lengthwise and across to make the "cubes".

Traditional Fries: If your sweet potato is large, cut it in half first. (This is not necessary for smaller potatoes.) Next, cut the whole or half potatoes into lengthwise wedges about 3/4 inch thick. You can stop here and roast large wedges, or you can cut the wedges further into smaller fries.

Coat with Oil & Balsamic Vinegar: Next, place the cubes into a bowl and drizzle with olive oil. (approximately 1 tablespoon). Don't drown them in oil. They should look glossy, but they shouldn't be sitting in a pool of olive oil. Optionally, if you want to bring out the sweetness of the potatoes, you can also drizzle a very small amount of Balsamic Vinegar over the potatoes right after you coat with the olive oil.

Add Seasonings & Mix: Season with a pinch of good quality sea salt and some pepper or with your favorite seasoning mix. (I usually use a seasoning blend that contains a variety of herbs and spices.) Combine all the ingredients, ensuring that all the potato cubes are well-coated.

Roast: Preheat the oven to 400°. (Some chefs roast at a little higher temperature, 425°. Try, both ways to see what works best for you.) Place the sweet potato cubes onto the baking sheet in a single layer. You can put a piece of parchment paper on the baking sheet, which makes cleanup easier. You can also use a Pyrex dish, but the higher the sides of the dish, the more the potatoes will "steam" instead of roasting. Also, avoid overcrowding the potatoes, as this will cause them to steam and become mushier on the outside. Bake for 30-45 minutes, turning every 10 minutes with spatula so that potatoes brown, but do not burn. Serve warm.

Janet's Sweet Potato Home Fries: Prepare roasted sweet potatoes. (You can prepare them ahead of time, refrigerate, and sauté the rest of the ingredients before serving**.**) Sauté chopped onions in a small amount of oil (I use olive oil or toasted sesame oil) until they are sweet and slightly browned. Then add chopped red and green peppers to the onions and sauté until the peppers are soft. Add in the sweet potatoes, and season with salt, pepper a (and if desired, a little garlic powder). Continue to sauté until the potatoes are warm and everything is mixed well together.

Versatile Kale Sides and Salads

Kale is a powerhouse vegetable, and is one of the highest-ranking vegetables on the ORAC scale. This is a rating that is based on a method of measuring the antioxidant capacity of fruits and vegetables. Foods are ranked according to their potential to mop up oxygen-free radicals. Choosing foods with a high ORAC value provides an extra nutritional boost. The top 10 ORAC scores per 4 oz. fresh produce include: blueberries, blackberries, garlic, kale, strawberries, spinach, Brussels sprouts, alfalfa sprouts, and broccoli. Kale contains seven times the beta carotene of broccoli and ten times as much lutein and zeaxanthin. These are eye protecting carotenoids that are known to protect against macular degeneration.

Kale can be lightly boiled, sautéed, or even used as a substitute for lettuce in salads.

Types of Kale:

Curly. Light green, curly-edged leaves with fibrous stems. Typically used in salads, slaws, soups, and prepared by roasting, blanching, sautéing, or steaming.

Lacinato (also known as Dinosaur Kale). Deep green, with flat elongated leaves and softer stems. The taste is sweeter and milder and is often used in soups, stews, and pasta.

Chinese Kale. Light green with large, glossy leaves and a thick stalk. Typically used in stir-fries.

Red Russian. Flat, broad leaves with a purple stem. The taste is mild, and the leaves are often used in salads

Baby Kale. Small, tender leaves. Baby kale is mild and sweet, and is used in salads, smoothies, or blanched or steamed.

Kale Serving Suggestions:

- Lightly boil (blanch) some kale, chop it up finely, and add it to some cooked grains. (such as barley or quinoa) For variety, add other chopped vegetables or sun-dried tomatoes.
- Add lightly boiled (blanched) chopped kale to your regular salad.
- Add chopped raw kale to winter soups such as minestrone
- Lightly sauté some chopped kale in olive oil. Add pine nuts and minced garlic for an extra layer of flavor. Eat as a side dish or add as an ingredient to pasta dishes.

- Prepare a lightly boiled, simple, warm kale salad. Chop finely and sprinkle with rice vinegar. For extra flavor, sprinkle some Gomashio over the kale. (a seasoning made of ground sesame seeds and other spices)
- Mix lightly boiled (blanched) chopped kale with finely chopped sauerkraut, coleslaw, or pressed red cabbage.
  - Substitute raw kale for romaine in Caesar Salad. For best results, lightly massage the Kale to make it less bitter, more tender, easier to chew, and more digestible.

How to Prepare Lightly Boiled (blanched) Kale:

Select the amount of kale appropriate for the dish you are making. (anywhere from a few leaves to an entire bunch of kale)

Wash kale well, checking on the underside of leaves for any grey/green aphids, which sometimes cling to kale leaves. If you are going to lightly boil the kale, there is no need to dry it. (When you sauté kale or use it in a salad, dry it well with a clean kitchen towel, paper towel, or use a salad spinner to dry the leaves.)

Either use your hands to strip the kale leaves off the stalk or use a knife to cut the leaves from the stalk. (If you want to use the stalks, you can prepare and cook them separately in boiling water and then chop them into small pieces. The stalks take a little longer to cook.)

Chop or tear the kale leaves into medium-sized pieces

Bring at least 2 cups of water to a boil. (more depending on the amount of kale you are boiling – the kale should be fully covered with water)

Blanch the kale by placing it into the water and if the water stops boiling, bring it back to a boil. Allow the kale to remain in the water until it turns a bright green color. (2-3 minutes) The point is to boil the kale until it is slightly tender. ***Do Not Overcook. If the kale cooks until it is dark green, it is overdone.***

Remove the kale from the water with a slotted spoon. To stop the kale from cooking further, immerse it in a bowl of cold water. Then, remove the mixture from the bowl and chop it into small pieces, using it in any of the recipes above.

Tips for Massaging Kale for Salads

Add a drizzle of olive oil: Add raw chopped kale to a large mixing bowl, and drizzle the leaves with a small amount of olive oil. (You can substitute avocado oil if desired.)

Massage the kale: Use clean hands to massage the kale with the oil (plus lemon or salt, if added) for 2-3 minutes to soften the leave and infuse the leaves with the oil. Towards the end of massaging, you can add other ingredients for additional flavor, such as a pinch of salt or touch of lemon juice. At the end of massaging, the kale should appear glossy and slightly reduced in volume.

Add to your favorite dishes: Once tenderized, your kale is ready to add to a salad or one of your other favorite recipes.

How to Make a Super Salad

Basic Preparation: Greens + Dressing + Veggies/Protein + Condiments

Use a variety of greens: There are many delicious and highly nutritious varieties of leafy greens available as an alternative to traditional iceberg lettuce. Try Arugula, Butterhead lettuce, Curly Endive, Mache, Mesclun, Romaine, Spinach, Watercress, or Kale for a flavorful salad that is rich in nutrients.

Add a variety of healthy vegetables and/or protein and condiments: Adding vegetables and/or protein and condiments such as nuts or seeds or cheese such as shaved parmesan or goat cheese makes your salad even more nutritious and provides a delicious balance of flavors and colors. Here are some ideas:

GREEN: Boston lettuce, Baby Spinach, Romaine, Watercress, Parsley, Mixed Field Greens, Arugula, Green Peppers, Chopped Kale, Pumpkin Seeds, Green Cabbage, Broccoli, Celery, Cucumber, Sprouts, Green Olives, Avocado.

YELLOW/ORANGE: Yellow Bell Pepper, Dried Apricot, Carrots, Mango, Sliced Orange, Small amounts of corn as a garnish, Pinto Beans.

BLUE/PURPLE: Blueberries, Red Grapes, Eggplant, Mission Figs, Blackberries, Arame (a type of sea vegetable often used as a salad ingredient in Japanese cuisine)

WHITE: Reduced Fat Goat Cheese, Jicama, Cauliflower, Firm Tofu, Mushrooms, Sunflower Seeds, Sesame Seeds, Garlic, Pine Nuts

RED: Tomatoes, Red Kidney Beans, Red Bell Pepper, Red Onion, Radicchio, Red Cabbage, Red Apple Slices, Red Onions, Sun Dried Tomatoes

Choose healthy oils for your salad dressings: Extra-virgin olive oil is a good choice. Try this simple recipe for a light, refreshing dressing: 1 tsp olive oil, ¼ cup lemon juice/ or lime juice, 2 tbs. chopped fresh parsley, 2 tbs. finely chopped onion, 1 clove garlic- finely chopped. Combine all ingredients and mix thoroughly. Add salt and pepper to taste.

Another foolproof way to "dress" your salad is to drizzle a small amount of extra-virgin olive oil over the greens and mix well. The greens should be lightly dressed, not soggy. Then add a small amount of your preferred vinegar or lemon juice to taste. Finally, add any seasonings and your veggies/protein and/or condiments.

Powerhouse Broccoli

Broccoli is a member of the Brassica family of cruciferous vegetables. broccoli is a great source of the vitamin C, folate, potassium, fiber, vitamin E and vitamin B6 all of which promote cardiovascular health

Broccoli Serving Suggestions:

- Puree leftover broccoli with some sautéed onions and mix with low-fat milk or almond milk with seasonings (try nutmeg) for a fast creamy soup
- Lightly steam or quick boil some broccoli and eat with low fat dip dressing
- Stir fry shredded cabbage (add onions for extra flavor)
- Roast broccoli, cauliflower with olive oil and a touch of balsamic vinegar
- Server raw or lightly steamed broccoli florets with hummus dip
- Sprinkle lemon juice and sesame seeds over lightly steamed broccoli
- Combine steamed quartered Brussels sprouts with sliced red onions, walnuts, and some mild-tasting cheese (such as feta). Toss with olive oil and balsamic vinegar for a light side dish.
- Sauté broccoli with red peppers, garlic and olive oil. (Dress with small of lemon)

Creamy Broccoli Salad:

INGREDIENTS: (makes 4 servings)

- 8 cups Broccoli (chopped into florets)
- 1/4 cup Red Onion (finely sliced)
- 1/4 cup Tahini
- 1 Lemon (juiced)
- 2 tbsps. Extra Virgin Olive Oil
- 1/4 tsp Sea Salt
- 1/4 tsp Black Pepper
- 2 tbsps. Water
- 1/3 cup Sunflower Seeds (plain Or Roasted

INSTRUCTIONS:

Bring a large pot of water to a boil and drop in your broccoli florets. Cover with a lid and boil for 2 - 3 minutes, or just until slightly tender. Strain and run under cold water.

Roughly chop the florets into pieces and add them to a large mixing bowl. Add in the red onion.

[Optional - Lightly marinate the red onion in red wine vinegar or other vinegar of choice before adding to the salad]

In a small to medium-sized bowl, combine the tahini, lemon juice, olive oil, sea salt, black pepper, and water, adding the water in small increments until the desired thickness is achieved.

Taste for flavor and serve as desired. Use less water for dips and sauces and more water for salad dressings. Pour over the salad and toss well.

OPTIONAL-ADD: 1/2 to 1 tablespoon white miso (to taste); 1/2 to 1 tablespoon tamari (or soy sauce to taste); pinch of red pepper flakes.

Sprinkle sunflower seeds over the top of the salad and serve.

Easy Pressed Red Cabbage:

Basic Preparation: Sliced Cabbage + Salt + Press + Rinse + Season [OPTIONAL Add Additional Vegetables/Condiments)

I learned how to make pressed salads while working as an apprentice to a macrobiotic chef. I never liked raw cabbage in salads, but pressed cabbage became a favorite. A pressed salad made with red or green cabbage is excellent for adding a crisp salad to meals, reducing sweet cravings, and satisfying the need for a crunchy texture. The beauty of pressing cabbage is that it brings out the sweetness of the cabbage and lends a deeper flavor to any dish.

The technique for making this salad is similar to making sauerkraut. Cabbage and other vegetables are sliced super thin and massaged with salt. A plate and a weight are placed on top, and the salad will sit, pressing for a period ranging from ½ hour to a few hours, depending on the desired texture and taste. The longer the salad is pressed, the softer the cabbage will become, and the longer the salt or other seasonings will have to infuse into the cabbage. The trick is to add enough sea salt or vinegar so that moisture is drawn out, but not so much that the cabbage becomes overly salty. When it is finished, there should be some liquid to pour off the salad, and some of the salt will go with it. After pouring off the excess liquid, if you find it is too salty, you can always rinse the cabbage to reduce the salty taste.

The recipe below is a basic pressed cabbage salad that can be eaten on its own or added to other dishes or stir-fries. You can dress it up by adding seeds, apples, or other shredded vegetables.

INGREDIENTS:

- ½ head red or green cabbage (or combination of both) (to make approximately 4-6 cups of sliced cabbage)
- ½ to 1 tsp sea salt (start small and add enough for moisture to be drawn from the cabbage) [Alternatively, you can use umeboshi paste or Ume vinegar instead of salt]
- OPTIONAL: 1-2 tsp vinegar of choice or lemon juice for additional flavor
- OPTIONAL: 1 tsp olive or sesame oil

- OPTIONAL: Additional thinly sliced vegetables

INSTRUCTIONS:

Slice the cabbage thinly lengthwise.

Place the cabbage in a large bowl and sprinkle with enough salt to draw water from it. Gently massage the salt into the cabbage. Continue until the cabbage begins to turn limp and release liquid. If you massage for a minute or two and the cabbage still feels dry, add a little more salt or Ume. (the salt removes water and acid from the cabbage)

Place a plate on top of the cabbage and weigh it down with something heavy that will press the plate down, such as a jar full of water or a heavy-filled can or container. The plate should cover the top of most of the salad without its edges contacting the sides of the bowl when pressing.

Allow the cabbage to sit in the bowl for approximately ½ hour to 1 hour until it is shiny and the desired tenderness.

Next, squeeze the cabbage gently between your hands to release the water and place it in a different bowl or plate. Or if desired, rinse cabbage lightly to remove most of the salt. Then drain & squeeze well. For additional flavor, combine the oil and vinegar of choice (or oil plus lemon juice) and pour over the cabbage and toss well. (For a lighter dressing, you can omit the olive oil)

OPTIONAL: Add additional thinly sliced vegetables, fruit, or top with seeds (pumpkin, sesame, sunflower) or sprinkle with Gomashio. Some suggested combinations:

- cabbage, daikon radish, cucumber, watercress
- cabbage, cucumber, red radish, parsley
- cabbage, green apple, red onion

Hearty Vegetable Soup

Once you understand the basics of soup, you can take any vegetable soup recipe and make it your own. You can also add a protein of choice, such as chicken, beans, or tofu, for a heartier soup. For a quick creamy soup, you can start with leftover cooked vegetables and add broth, coconut milk or 1/2 and ½ and use an immersion or regular blender to blend it until it is a smooth consistency. When pressed for time, you can start with a combination of already cooked or frozen vegetables, prepared broth or stock, and seasonings to create a quick, on-the-spot vegetable soup. In the morning, I often combine sautéed shiitake mushrooms, onions, and tofu with a container of turmeric/ginger flavored chicken bone broth for a hearty breakfast.

Basic Preparation: Soup Base + Seasonings + Broth + Vegetables + (Optional Protein) + Garnish

1. Prepare the Base.

Great soups start with a combination of aromatic vegetables cooked in oil to bring out their flavor. To start, heat 2 TBSPS extra-virgin olive oil in a large pot over medium heat.

Next add 1 cup diced vegetables of choice. (This traditionally includes onions, celery, carrots which is the traditional "Mirepoix" ---- the French culinary term for a combination of diced carrots, onions and celery sautéed in oil or butter and used as an aromatic base to flavor sauces, soups and stews.) You can use one or all, whatever you have on hand. (Make it fast tip: You can purchase Mirepoix chopped and ready to go at most grocery stores)

If you want the soup to have a garlic flavor, you can add some minced garlic to the diced vegetables. (Make it fast tip: purchase pre-made mirepoix and pre-minced garlic)

Stir the vegetables in the oil until softened. (2-3 minutes)

2. Season.

Add seasonings to the diced vegetables and stir for 1-2 minutes more. The easiest thing is to use a Seasoning Mix (I like Trader Joe's 21 Salute) if you are going for a classic vegetable soup or you can make your own combination of seasonings.

At this point, my rule of thumb is to go light on the seasonings, now and then later taste the soup and add more as needed. The types of seasonings you add depends on the desired end result. Want your soup extra spicy? Red Pepper Flakes are an option. Want more of a Japanese Vegetable Soup? You might add some ginger and miso. Going for Mexican? Chipotle chilies might be a good addition.

3. Add the Broth or Stock.

Generally, a good amount is 4 cups of liquid (or 8 cups for a larger batch)

You can start with boxed or canned broth or stock or prepare your own broth from scratch.

On special occasions I prepare my own broth, but for the most part I like to start with a well-prepared packaged bone or vegetable broth. Buying a low-sodium versions allow you to control the seasoning of your soup while also cutting back on the salt content. Depending on the flavoring you desire and whether you want your soup to be vegetarian. there are many different options to choose from.

NOTE: If you are going to use "uncooked" chicken or other meat, add it to the broth now, and simmer until cooked through. Then remove from the broth and cut up or shred to add back into the soup at the end. If you are going for "easy" use already cooked meat or poultry that can be shredded/cubed and added at the end.

4. Add Vegetables. (they can be fresh or frozen) (2-6 Cups depending on amount of broth)

Make it fast tip: Use frozen or pre-cut veggies

You can pick your vegetables based on what you have on hand, or the type of flavor you want. Below are some suggested vegetables by color

- WHITE: Rutabaga, Turnips, White Cabbage, Cauliflower
- ORANGE: Carrots, Winter Squash, Sweet Potato
- GREEN: Kale, Spinach, Broccoli, Chard, Collards, Green Beans, Celery, Zucchini, Peas
- BROWN: Mushrooms (button, shitake, porcini, portobello)
- PURPLE: Purple Cabbage, Eggplant
- YELLOW: Yellow Squash, Corn
- RED: Tomatoes (canned or fresh)

Simmer the vegetables until vegetables are tender. 5-15 minutes.

Taste, and add any additional seasonings, as desired. (and if desired Add Protein – Step #5) and simmer the vegetables and protein together.

5. ADD PROTEIN (if desired)

You can add cooked chicken (cubed or shredded) or beans (Black Beans, Cannellini, Chick Peas, Kidney Beans, Navy Beans), tofu or seafood such as cooked shrimp.

If you are adding beans, the easiest is to use canned/rinsed beans or leftover cooked beans.

6. ADD A FINAL LAYER OF FLAVOR

Ever wonder why restaurant soups taste so good. One secret is adding a "pop" of flavor at the end bring all the flavors together and add depth to the overall taste. There are several ways to do this.

Add something Acidic like a touch of lemon, lime or vinegar. The trick here is to start with a very small amount (1/4 tsp) and taste. The soup should not taste vinegary or like lemon or lime. The purpose is just to add enough to bring out all the flavors of the soup.

For a more "umami" taste, you can add a small amount of fish sauce, miso or tamari. Again, a very small amount to add richness, not salty taste)

For a more complex taste, you could also top with some pesto, curry paste or sriracha if you want to add some heat or herb flavoring. A sprinkling of fresh herbs is always a nice final addition

Easy Baked Salmon

I love fish, but I am not a big fan of cooking it. So, I keep it pretty simple. Salmon is one of my favorite options, and I usually try to buy one of the wild salmon varieties. A really easy way to prepare delicious salmon with great results is to bake it with a simple, no-sugar-added marinade. There are lots of bottled options, or you can create your own.

Basic Preparation: Select Salmon + Prepare Marinade + Apply Marinade & Seasonings + Bake

STEP #1: SELECT SALMON

There are two broad categories of salmon: farmed salmon and wild salmon. Wild salmon are captured by fishing vessels from their natural habitat, whereas farmed salmon are bred and harvested in controlled water environments.

Since there is no seafood labeling system in place at fish markets, fish counters of grocery stores, and restaurants that serve fresh seafood, if you want to know more about the fish you are buying, some of the questions you can ask include:

- What country is the fish from?
- Is the fish wild-caught or farm-raised?
- If it is farmed, was it grown in an open net pen or a closed system

There are several species of wild Pacific salmon, each differing slightly in taste, texture, color, and nutritional value, including:

Chinook/King: The largest—and often most expensive—the king or chinook is prized for its high-fat content and buttery texture.

Sockeye/Red: An oilier fish with deep red flesh, sockeye salmon has a stronger flavor and stands up well to grilling.

Coho/Silver: Coho is milder and often lighter in color.

Humpback/Pink and Keta/Chum: These smaller salmon are most often used for canned or smoked salmon. They're also good budget choices.

Several countries produce farmed salmon, including Norway, Chile, Scotland, and North America. Fish farming industries in all these countries are highly regulated, although the quality can vary based on various factors including the type of fish feed used, use of antibiotics, and the method of farming.

Atlantic salmon are anadromous fish, meaning they are born in freshwater, migrate to the ocean to grow, and return to freshwater to reproduce. They were once an abundant species, but today, due to overfishing and other environmental factors, they are now an endangered species, and commercial and recreational fishing for

Atlantic salmon in the United States is prohibited. Atlantic Salmon is commercially available exclusively through farm-raised production.

Farm-raised Norwegian salmon is known for its mild flavor and delicate texture. Their cold, clean waters are ideal for farming healthy and flavorful fish.

Chilean farmed salmon is known for its rich flavor and firm texture. The country has made significant strides in improving sustainability practices in recent years.

Scottish farmed salmon is known for its rich flavor and buttery texture.

STEP #2: Prepare the Salmon

Skin On or Off? Many prefer to cook salmon with the skin on because it helps retain moisture during cooking, resulting in juicier and more tender flesh. Additionally, the skin acts as a protective layer, keeping the flesh intact. If you are baking, frying, searing, or grilling salmon, this fatty layer helps prevent the fish from becoming overcooked. If you leave the skin on during cooking, you can remove it before serving by sliding a spatula between the skin and the flesh. This will leave the salmon skin on the baking sheet or cooking pan. Another method is to place the cooked salmon skin-side up on a plate or cutting board. Using a fork, gently pull the skin off the fillet.

If you prefer to cook salmon without the skin, the con is that you need to master a method of removing the skin before cooking. The skin can sometimes result in an oily or fishy flavor that might not suit everyone's palate. Without the skin, seasoning and marinating can penetrate the flesh more thoroughly, enhancing the overall flavor. Also, it is best to poach salmon with the skin removed.

STEP #3: PREPARE MARINADE

The basic preparation for marinades: Healthy fat + Acid + Seasoning + Spices

- Fats include: Olive oil, Avocado oil, Full-fat coconut milk,
- Acids include: Vinegar (apple cider, rice, wine, or any other type), Citrus juice (lemon, lime, orange),

- Seasonings include: Coconut aminos, Tamari, Soy sauce, Mustard, Worcestershire sauce, Fish sauce, Sriracha sauce, Sugar-Free Maple Syrup or Honey, Sweeteners of choice (such as Stevia, Monk Fruit, or Allulose)
- Spices include: Minced/pressed garlic or ginger, chili flakes, herbs (fresh or dry), salt, pepper

Preparing, Tasting, and Handling Marinades:

- Whisk together all marinade ingredients in a small bowl or jar.
- Taste your marinade and adjust your seasonings before adding to your fish – some seasonings and acids pack more punch than others.
- Do not taste marinades after adding them to raw fish or meat.
- Do not reuse marinade that has been poured over raw fish or meat. If you want to reserve some for basting or serving, set aside some of the marinade in a bowl or jar before pouring it over your fish for later use.
- Don't marinate salmon at room temperature. Refrigeration is vital for food safety with raw seafood.

Sample Marinades:

Asian: 1-2 Tbsp Olive oil, 1-2 Tbsp Lime juice, 2 tbsp Fresh parsley, 1 tbsp Fresh dill, 1 clove Garlic (minced), 1 tbsp tamari, soy sauce or coconut aminos, 1/4 tsp Black pepper

Chili Lime: 1 TBSP Olive Oil, ¼ tsp pepper, ¼ tsp salt, ½ tsp chili powder, ½ tsp garlic powder, 1-2 TBSP Lime Juice, and ½ TBSP Lime Zest (Optional).

Lemon Dill: 1-2 tbsp melted grass-fed butter or ghee (you can substitute olive oil if desired), 1-2 cloves minced garlic, 2 tbsp fresh dill, 1 lemon juiced & zested ¼, ¼ tsp, and sea salt.

Sesame Ginger: 2 Tbsp sesame oil, 2 Tbsp olive oil, 2 Tbsp coconut aminos, Dash of chili pepper or your favorite hot sauce, 2-3 Tbsp rice vinegar, 1½ Tbsp sugar free maple syrup or other sweetener of choice, 2 cloves garlic, finely minced, 1 Tbsp freshly minced ginger

STEP #4: Marinate the Salmon

Marinating salmon significantly enhances its flavor without compromising the inherent great taste of the fish. The marinating time will depend on the type of salmon, the cut/size (cubes, filets, steaks, or whole), and the specific marinade used. Acidity and salt break down salmon's delicate flesh. Unlike red meat, salmon is best marinated for no more than 1-2 hours, or ½ hour when applying more acidic marinades, such as a lemon-based.

Place the salmon in the marinade using either a shallow dish or a Ziplock bag.

Dish Method: Place the salmon in a shallow dish large enough to fit all your salmon pieces side by side. You may need to use several dishes if you are doubling or tripling the recipe. Pour the marinade over the fish, ensuring it is fully covered. Turn the fish a couple of times to ensure each side is evenly covered. Let it marinate in the refrigerator for ½ hour (more acidic marinades) or 1-2 hours.

Ziplock Bag Method: Place the salmon in a large zip-top plastic bag, then pour in the marinade. Seal the bag and massage the fish to coat the salmon evenly. (Press out as much air as possible before sealing the bag.) Place the bag on a large plate and refrigerate for ½ hour (for more acidic marinades) or 1-2 hours.

STEP #4: Bake the Salmon

Preheat Oven: While researching and preparing recipes, I have found that recommended cooking temperatures for salmon vary significantly, ranging from 350°F to 400°F. Many chefs swear by the method of cooking fast at a higher temperature for a moister result. Others recommend a lower temperature and a slower-bake method. The main thing is to watch the salmon closely at the end so that it does not overcook. When baking salmon, I typically set the oven temperature to 350°F. (You can experiment to determine your preference.)

Remove the fish from the marinade. Discard the liquid that the fish was marinating in. If you wish to pour some marinade over the fish while it is baking, use some of the prepared marinade that you set aside for this purpose.

Transfer the fish to a prepared baking dish or a baking sheet.

Place the salmon in the baking dish or baking sheet, skin-side down, leaving sufficient space between each piece to ensure even cooking.

Choose whether to use parchment paper, aluminum foil, or a lightly greased dish or baking sheet. Using parchment paper or aluminum foil will prevent the salmon from sticking and make cleanup easier. If using aluminum foil, you can gently fold the edges of the foil up to seal the fish in a pouch. This method yields a very moist and flaky result.

If desired, you can add spices, herbs, lemon slices, or vegetables for extra flavor before baking.

Bake the salmon until done. At 350 degrees, the fish generally needs to cook for 20-25 minutes. However, it's best to check it at around 15 minutes to ensure it's not drying out. At higher temperatures, 12-15 minutes is a good guide. The cooking time will vary depending on the type of salmon, the thickness, and the desired level of doneness. Wild Salmon is more prone to becoming dry and overcooked, as it generally has less fat than farmed salmon.

Check for doneness by inserting a fork or knife into the thickest part of the salmon. If it flakes easily, it's done. You can also use an instant-read thermometer to test for doneness. Insert the thermometer into the thickest portion of the fish. According to the FDA, salmon should be cooked to an internal temperature of 145°F. At a lower temperature, the salmon will be medium-rare, and cooking to 145 will provide a more well-done result.

Before serving, if you want the top of the salmon to be a bit crispy, place it under the broiler for a few moments. Also, a nice flavor addition is to garnish the fully cooked salmon with lemon and/or lime slices.

SUGAR-FREE PUDDINGS & CREAMY DESSERTS

Sometimes I crave something sweet, but I need to stay away from baked goods, even if they are made with sugar alternatives. Creamy no-bake puddings are satisfying, easy to make, and sugar alternatives blend well into pudding mixtures. Ideas for different puddings are almost endless. Below are a few suggestions.

Creamy Yogurt Puddings

Nothing is easier than jazzing up yogurt to satisfy a sweet tooth. There is no need to consume brands with lots of added sugar or aspartame, when you can so easily make your own creations. Both Greek and Icelandic brands serve as the perfect base for a creamy pudding. Experiment with flavors and sweeteners to find your favorite.

For a chocolate "pudding," add the following (with amounts to taste) to plain Greek or Icelandic yogurt: Cacao powder, chocolate whey powder, and sweetener of choice. I generally add approximately 1 tsp of cacao powder, ½ scoop of chocolate whey powder, and chocolate liquid stevia to taste.

For a more decadent treat, mix in a tablespoon of melted sugar-free chocolate and top with a swirl of whipped cream.

Ricotta Pudding Whips

Ricotta puddings have been a go-to snack for me since I was first diagnosed, and I "jazz" them up based on my mood at the time.

The basic recipe is ½ cup half-skim Ricotta + flavoring of choice + Sweetener of Choice. (Example, Ricotta, plus Vanilla Extract, plus Splenda or Stevia). You mix all the ingredients, chill, and enjoy. I generally mix with a spoon, but you could also combine the ingredients in a food processor.

Additional Options:

Add Vanilla Whey Powder to the combination above. (You can also include some whipped cream or a small amount of mascarpone for extra creaminess.)

Add in a ¼ -½ teaspoon of bottled cold brew coffee and a small amount of plain or espresso-flavored mascarpone for a coffee-flavored treat.

Mix in sugar-free chocolate chips to create a Ricotta Cannoli Cup recipe

Mix in some pureed pumpkin and pumpkin pie spice for a delicious pumpkin pie pudding.

-

APPENDIX B
Suggested Reading and Resources

Navigating Change and Decluttering

The Power of Now: Eckhart Tolle, New World Library, 1999. Conquering sugar and any chronic illness such as diabetes requires living in the present moment. If you are stuck in the past, moving forward will be almost impossible. Worrying about the future and what could happen can immobilize you. The Power of Now provides excellent insights on how to make the most of today.

The Four Agreements: A Practical Guide to Personal Freedom: Don Miguel Ruiz, Amber-Allen Publishing, 1997. In this timeless book, you will uncover the origins of self-limiting beliefs that hinder our joy and shape our reality. Based on ancient Toltec wisdom, *The Four Agreements* offers a path that can transform your life so that you can experience freedom from sabotaging behaviors and enjoy vibrant physical, mental, and spiritual well-being.

If emotional eating is an issue for you, the three books below can open the door to changing long-standing beliefs and modifying your behaviors. You will gain a deeper understanding of how to cultivate awareness, enabling you to transform your belief system and develop a more balanced relationship with food.

The Power of Belief: Ray Dodd, Hampton Roads Publishing Co., Inc., 2003.

The Miracle of Mindfulness: Thich Nhat Hanh, Beacon Press Books, 1976

Eating Mindfully: Susan Albers, psy.d., New Harbinger Publications, Inc., 2003.

The Life-Changing Magic of Tidying Up, Marie Kondo, Ten Speed Press, 2014. Japanese cleaning consultant Marie Kondo offers a novel approach to simplify and organize your home with a category-by-category system. While some prefer traditional room-by-room decluttering techniques, her book explores how maintaining only what sparks joy in your home fosters an environment that helps you achieve results in all areas of your life.

Diabetes and Diabetes Management

Reversing Diabetes, by Julian Whitaker, M.D., Warner Books Inc., 1987, revised 2001. Filled with excellent insights and information, anyone with diabetes will come away with a deeper understanding of this chronic disease and practical ideas for managing it effectively.

Dr. Bernstein's Diabetes Solution, by Richard K. Bernstein, M.D., Little Brown Publishing, 1997. Not everyone will be able to adopt all of the recommendations provided by Dr. Bernstein. However, if you are serious about managing your diabetes, you will gain valuable insights into the nature of the disease and how to manage your blood sugar levels on a day-to-day basis.

Food & Nutrition

Get the Sugar Out, by Ann Louis Gittleman, Three Rivers Press, 1996. There is no doubt about it, giving up sugar is not easy. A classic and forerunner to newer books about the pitfalls of sugar, there are so many good ideas in this book for eliminating sugar and substituting with other satisfying foods, you might find you don't miss sugar after all.

The End of Overeating: David A. Kessler, M.D., Rodale, Inc., 2009. Dr. Kessler's book unlocks the mysteries of why many people struggle with overeating. Dr. Kessler explains why we overeat when we consume foods that contain sugar, fat, and salt, especially when these ingredients found in abundance in processed foods are manipulated in a certain way to stimulate our appetites.

Against all Grain: Danielle Walker, Victory Belt Publishing, Inc., 2013. Danielle Walker's cookbook is a treasure trove of delicious recipes that will help you avoid missing grains if you choose to cut back for improved blood sugar control. Her book features over 150 recipes that are entirely grain-free, gluten-free, free of refined sugars, and low to minimal in dairy.

Vegetarian Cooking for Everyone: Deborah Madison, Broadway Books, 1997. If you're not accustomed to eating a lot of vegetables and whole grains, preparing them in a variety of ways can be intimidating. The winner of prestigious awards such as the James Beard Foundation Award for Excellence, the recipes in this book will make a vegetable lover out of anyone.

Get Cooking, Molly Katzen, The Harper Studio, 2009. The cover of this cookbook says it all: "150 simple recipes to get you started in the kitchen." If you're looking to learn how to prepare healthy meals in your own kitchen, this book will help you transition from ordering out to making delicious foods at home.

The Sweet Life: Diabetes without Boundaries: Sam Talbot, Rodale Press, 2011. Beautifully written and photographed, this is one of my favorite recipe books. Sam's message is that you don't have to give up eating well. If you enjoy good food, you'll find plenty of options in these nutrient-rich recipes.

How to Cook Without a Book, Completely Updated and Revised: Recipes and Techniques Every Cook Should Know by Heart: Pam Anderson, Clarkson Potter, 2018. Pam Anderson's book is an excellent guide for anyone looking to go sugar-free and master easy techniques for creating simple, delicious meals. Understanding that most recipes are variations on a theme, Pam teaches a cooking style that enables you to use recipes as a guide, allowing you to create dishes that work for your sugar-free lifestyle.

The Joy of Gluten-Free Sugar Free Baking: Peter Reinhart & Demine Wallace, Ten Speed Press, 2012. If you enjoy a treat now and then and are looking for grain-free and sugar-free baking recipes, this book is for you. The delicious and easy-to-follow recipes can teach you how to use ingredients and create baked goods that come out perfectly, even if you are not an expert baker.

APPENDIX C
Worksheets

I have compiled the key worksheets used throughout each chapter for multiple use, easy copying, and downloading.

You can also find out how to access worksheets, workbooks, recipes, daily journals, and other resources on our website at www.sugarfreelifestylecoaching.com.

Change Readiness Assessment

How often do you agree with each statement below?	Never	Rarely	Sometimes	Always
Pre-Contemplation. "I don't see a need for change in my relationship with sugar."				
Contemplation. "I know I should change, and I am thinking about it, but there are things about sugar I like. I am not sure what I want to change."				
Preparation. "I am ready to change and adopt a sugar-free lifestyle, but I don't know how to move forward. I need a plan."				
Action. "I am ready to change and take action, although I know challenges may be ahead."				
Maintenance. "I am keeping up with my behavior changes, although it is not always easy."				
Relapse. "I make some decisions that lead me away from my goals. I need to reflect, adjust, and take action to get back on track."				

Food Assessment

	Item	Optimal Recommendation	Rating	Rating Description
Eat More	Non-starchy Vegetables	1-2 Servings each Meal/ Snack		**GREEN:** I consume 5-7 Days a week **YELLOW:** I eat occasionally. **RED:** I rarely consume
	Healthy Protein	1 Serving each Meal/ Snack		
	Healthy Fats	1 Serving each Meal/ Snack		
Avoid Or Eliminate	Added Sugar	Eliminate*		**GREEN:** I rarely consume **YELLOW:** I eat 3-5 times a week **RED:** I eat often or every day *Added sugar less than 1 gram OK on occasion, unless any added sugar is a trigger food.
	White Potatoes	Avoid		
	Grain-based flour products	Eliminate		
	Rice	White Rice (Eliminate)		
		Brown Rice (Avoid)		
	Soda	Regular Soda (Eliminate)		
		Diet Soda (Avoid)		
	Fruit	High Glycemic (Eliminate)		
		Medium Glycemic (Avoid)		
		Low Glycemic (Consume Sparingly)		
	Whole Grains	Quinoa (Consume Occasionally)		
		Other Grains (Avoid or consume in small portions occasionally		
	Starchy Vegetables	Consume in small portions occasionally.		

Trigger Food Worksheet

Trigger Food Motivators	Description	My Trigger Foods
Convenience & Ultra-Processed Foods	What foods with added sugar, hidden sugar, or high natural sugar do you eat/buy because of their convenience?	
Habit	What foods with added sugar, hidden sugar, or high natural sugar do you eat out of habit?	Breakfast: Lunch: Dinner: Other:
Life Situations	List 3 life situations that motivate you to eat trigger foods. What trigger foods do you eat in those situations?	
HALT	What trigger foods do you eat if you let yourself become too Hungry, Angry, Lonely, or Tired?	H: A: L: T:
Emotional Eating	List 3-4 emotions that motivate you to eat trigger foods. What trigger foods do you eat when you feel these emotions?	

Lifestyle Assessment: Defined

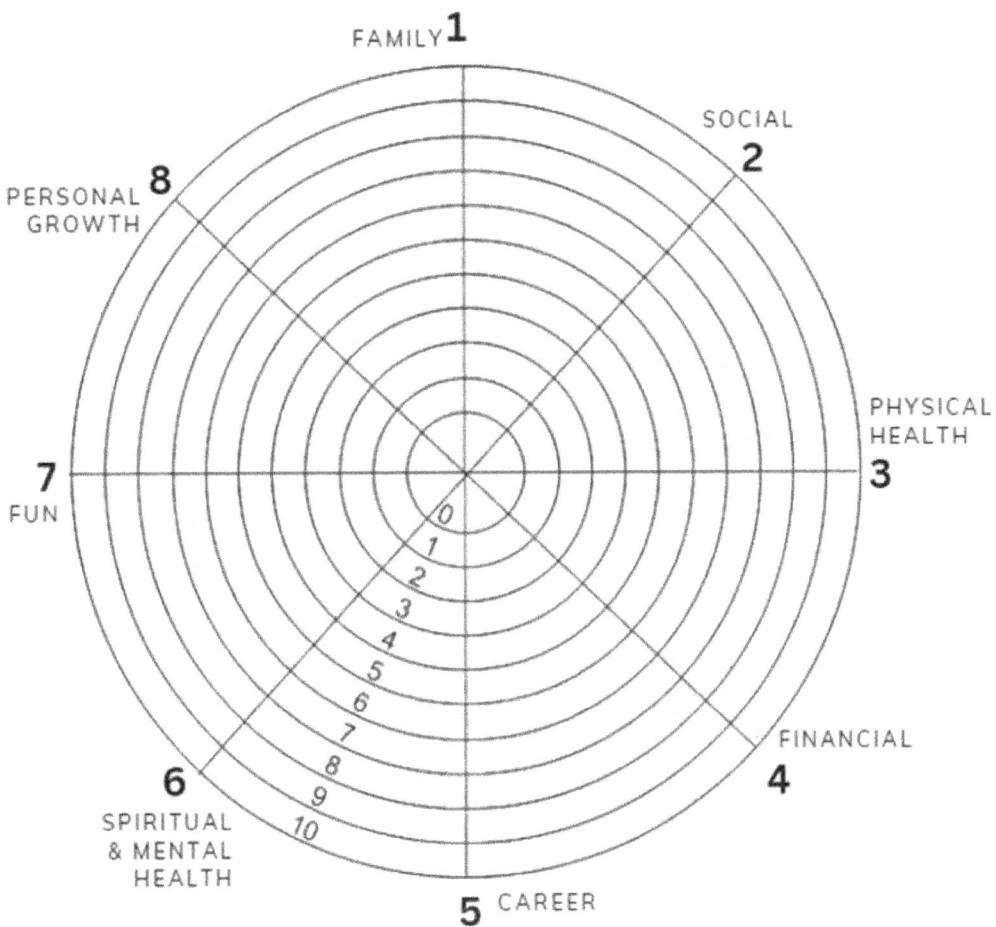

Lifestyle Assessment: Self-Defined

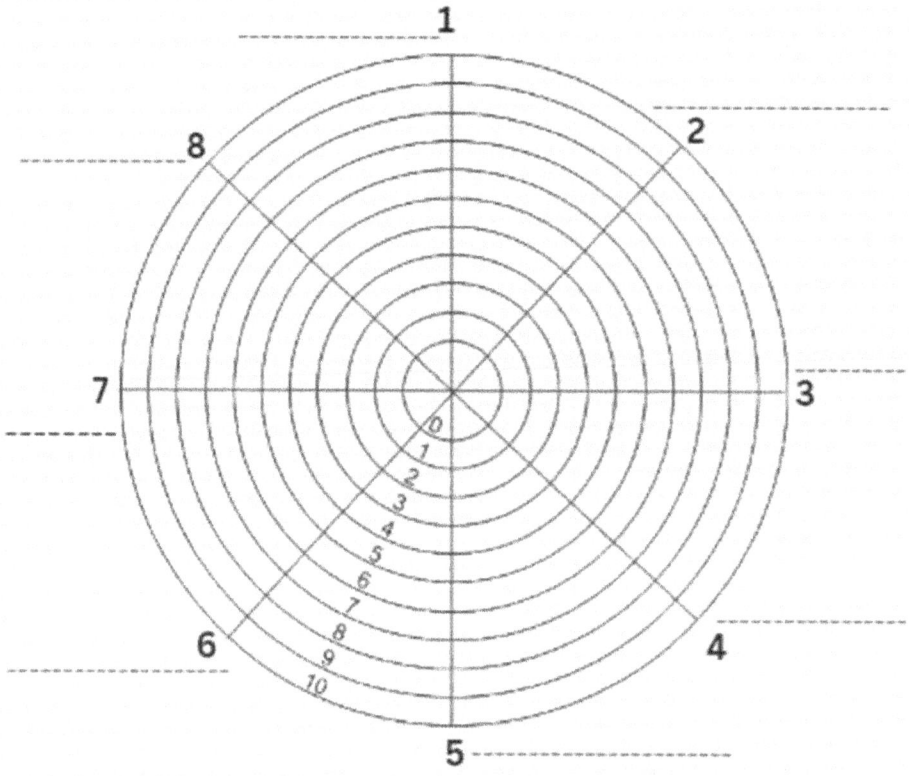

List the Categories that are most significant to you and use those for your Wheel of Life Assessment.

1)_____
2)_____
3)_____
4)_____
5)_____
6)_____
7)_____
8)_____

Feelings/Emotions Assessment

Feelings	Never	Rarely	Occasionally	Often	Every Day
Angry					
Anxious					
Depressed					
Deprived					
Nervous					
Sad					
Tired					
Worried					
Calm					
Confident					
Energized					
Excited					
Hopeful					
Joyful					
Peaceful					
Proud					
Other:					

Vision Exercise

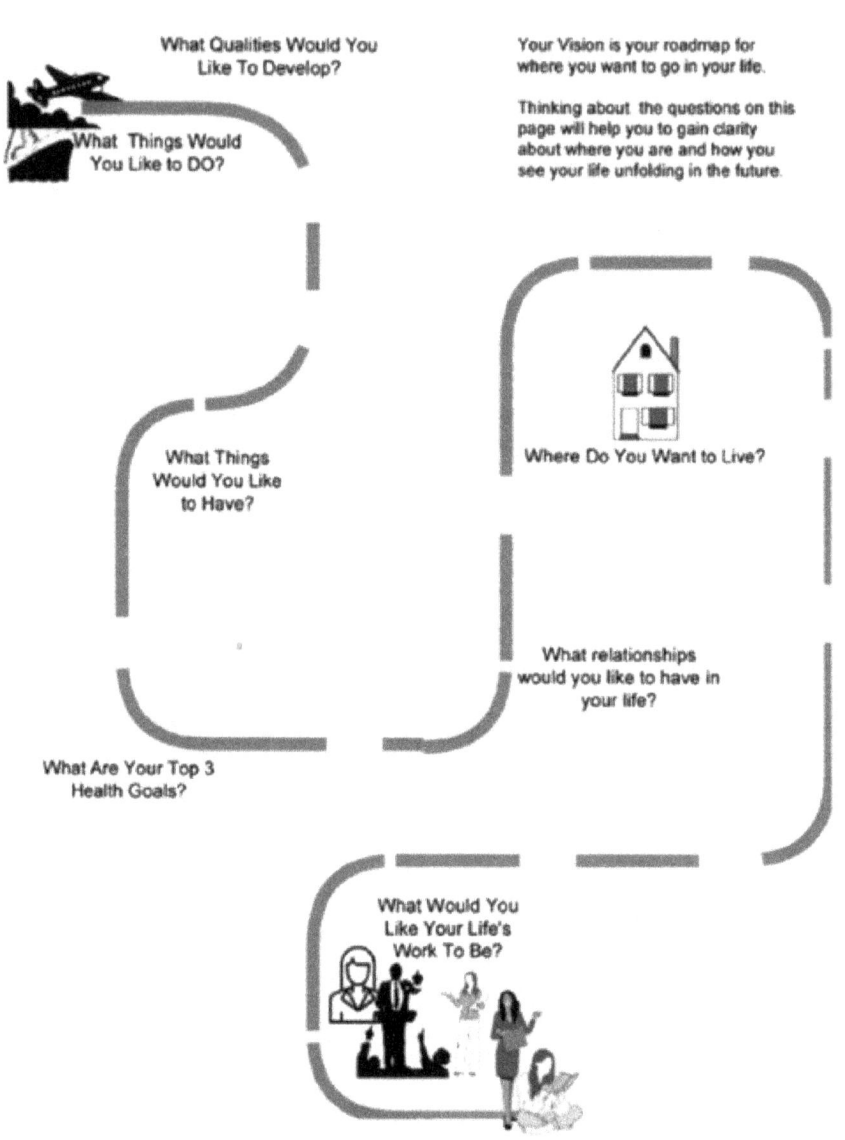

Short Term & Long-Term Goal Setting Worksheet

	Short/Long Term Goals
1 Month Goals	
3 Month Goals	
6 Month Goals	
1 Year Goals	
5 Year Goals	
Lifetime Goals	

Action Plan Worksheet

	Action Plan (Goal/Sub-Goals/Activities)
GOAL	
Sub-Goal #1	
• SG#1 Activities	
• SG#1 Obstacles & Solutions	
Sub-Goal #2	
• SG#2 Activities	
• SG#2 Obstacles & Solutions	
Sub-Goal #3	
• SG#3 Activities	
• SG#3 Obstacles & Solutions	

7 Day Meal Plan

	Breakfast	Lunch	Dinner
Day 1			
Day 2			
Day 3			
Day 4			
Day 5			
Day 6			
Day 7			

21 Day Habit Tracker

Write the new habit you have committed to in the box below, along with any notes or activities you have identified to help you perform this habit.

Place an X in the circles below on each day that you put your new habit into place. If you miss a day, leave a blank circle and place a check the next time you perform the habit
START DATE:

Sunday	Monday	Tuesday	Wednesday	Thursday	Friday	Saturday
○	○	○	○	○	○	○
○	○	○	○	○	○	○
○	○	○	○	○	○	○
○	○	○	○	○	○	○

Daily Food Tracker

FOOD TRACKER
DATE:

25% HIGH QUALITY PROTEIN
50% NON-STARCHY VEGETABLES
25% OTHER*

BREAKFAST
TIME:

Cross out 1 bottle for each Serving of Water Consumed
1 bottle = 8 ounces

LUNCH
TIME:

DINNER
TIME:

Blood Sugar Testing Results:

Time:
Result:

SNACKS
TIME(S):

Time:
Result:

Time:
Result:

TODAY, I AM GRATEFUL FOR:

"Stress Busters"
1 heart = 15 minutes

Exercise
1 figure = 1/2 hr

Weekly Crowd Out Tracker

	SUN	MON	TUE	WED	THU	FRI	SAT
ADDED SUGAR							
No beverages with added sugar							
No soda with added sugar							
(No diet soda)							
No recipes with added sugar							
No salad dressings with added sugar							
No processed foods with added sugar							
No yogurt with added sugar							
No high fructose corn syrup							
No yogurt with added sugar							
HIDDEN SUGAR							
No Grain-Based flour bread							
No Grain-Based flour crackers, muffins, tortillas, cookies, cakes, snacks							
No white potatoes							
No wheat-based pasta (small amounts of high protein, wheat mixed with lupini bean flour, or other types of wheat pasta alternatives OK)							
NO or very small portion of whole grains (Small amount of steel-cut oats, barley, quinoa OK)							
FRUIT, DAIRY, NATURAL SUGAR							
No high glycemic fruit (a small piece of non-ripe banana is OK in a smoothie)							
If desired, consume medium/low glycemic fruit sparingly.							
If desired, consume lactose dairy or lactose-free dairy products in moderation.							

www.ingramcontent.com/pod-product-compliance
Lightning Source LLC
Chambersburg PA
CBHW061819290426
44110CB00027B/2917